The Atypical Stutterer
Principles and Practices of Rehabilitation

SPEECH, LANGUAGE, AND HEARING
A Series of Monographs and Texts

Norman J. Lass
Department of Speech Pathology and Audiology
West Virginia University
Morgantown, West Virginia

A complete list of titles in this series is available from the publisher.

The Atypical Stutterer
Principles and Practices of Rehabilitation

Edited by

KENNETH O. ST. LOUIS

Speech Pathology and Audiology
West Virginia University
Morgantown, West Virginia

1986

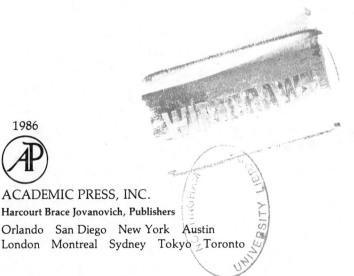

ACADEMIC PRESS, INC.
Harcourt Brace Jovanovich, Publishers
Orlando   San Diego   New York   Austin
London   Montreal   Sydney   Tokyo   Toronto

306001

ACADEMIC PRESS, INC.
Orlando, Florida 32887

United Kingdom Edition published by
ACADEMIC PRESS INC. (LONDON) LTD.
24–28 Oval Road, London NW1 7DX

LIBRARY OF CONGRESS CATALOGING-IN-PUBLICATION DATA

Main entry under title:

The Atypical stutterer.

   Includes index.
   1. Stuttering—Patients—Rehabilitation.
I. St. Louis, Kenneth O.
RC424.A82   1985   616.85′54   85-11058
ISBN 0-12-661620-5 (alk. paper)
ISBN 0-12-661621-3 (paperback)

PRINTED IN THE UNITED STATES OF AMERICA

86 87 88 89   9 8 7 6 5 4 3 2 1

This volume is dedicated to those stutterers who so willingly place their individual futures in our hands. May we never take that trust lightly or cease our striving to remain worthy of it.

Contents

Contributors   xi

Preface   xiii

CHAPTER 1
The Problem of the Atypical Stutterer: An Introduction   1
Kenneth O. St. Louis

    Purpose   1
    Some Troublesome Issues   3
    References   7

CHAPTER 2
Treating the Stutterer with Atypical Cultural Influences   9
William R. Leith

    Cultures in the United States   9
    Development of Stuttering: Cultural Influences   12
    Treatment of Stuttering: Cultural Influences   18
    Resources for Clinicians   29
    References and Recommended Readings   33

CHAPTER 3
The Female Stutterer   35
Ellen-Marie Silverman

    Introduction   35
    Female Stutterers   37

Assessment Strategies   45
Treatment   53
The Challenge of the Female Stutterer   59
References   60

CHAPTER 4
The Exceptionally Severe Stutterer   65
Pat Richard Sacco

Introduction   65
Definition of Stuttering   66
Characteristics of the Exceptionally Severe Stutterer   67
Distribution of Stuttering Severity in the General Population   68
Other Characteristics   70
Attitudinal Measures   72
Speech Rate and Prosody   74
Diagnostic Considerations   74
Treatment Rationale   76
Commitment to Treatment   83
The Triad of Treatment   83
Dismissal from Formal Treatment   86
Treatment Summary   87
Training Perspectives   88
References   89

CHAPTER 5
The Psychologically Maladjusted Stutterer   93
Michael D. Cox

Introduction   93
Description of the Psychologically Maladjusted Stutterer   94
Descriptive Studies   96
Psychoanalytic Contributions   96
Identification of Maladjustment   110
Treatment Considerations   114
Supportive Therapy   115
Group Therapy   118
Family Therapy   119
Summary   120
References   121

CHAPTER 6
The Mentally Retarded Stutterer   123
Eugene B. Cooper

The Mentally Retarded   124
Prevalence of Stuttering in the Mentally Retarded   126

The Nature of Stuttering in the Mentally Retarded   128
Diagnostic Considerations   134
Therapy with the Mentally Retarded Stutterer   143
Summary   151
References   152

CHAPTER 7
The Clutterer   155
David A. Daly

Cluttering Defined   156
Description and Characteristics   158
Comparisons between Cluttering and Stuttering   172
Assessment Procedures   175
Therapeutic Considerations   179
Case Studies   183
Summary   187
References   188

CHAPTER 8
Diagnosis and Management of Neurogenic Stuttering in Adults   193
Nancy Helm-Estabrooks

Introduction   193
Varieties of Neurogenic Stuttering   194
Diagnosis and Assessment of Neurogenic Stuttering   203
Management of Neurogenic Stuttering   207
Summary   211
Appendix 1: Guide to Differential Diagnosis of Neurogenic
     Stuttering   212
Appendix 2: Kalotkin Protocol: Relaxation Training for Treatment
     of Stuttering   213
References   215

Author Index   219
Subject Index   225

Contributors

Numbers in parentheses indicate the pages on which the authors' contributions begin.

Eugene B. Cooper (123), Department of Communicative Disorders, University of Alabama, University, Alabama 35486

Michael D. Cox (93), Psychology Division, Department of Psychiatry, Baylor College of Medicine, Houston, Texas 77037

David A. Daly (155), Department of Communication Disorders, University of Michigan, Ann Arbor, Michigan 48109

Nancy Helm-Estabrooks (193), Neurology Service, Boston Veterans Administration Hospital, and Boston University School of Medicine, Boston, Massachusetts 02130

William R. Leith (9), Speech and Language Center, Wayne State University, Detroit, Michigan 48202

Pat Richard Sacco (65), Speech and Hearing Clinics, State University of New York at Geneseo, Geneseo, New York 14454

Ellen-Marie Silverman[1] (35), Communication Disorders Curriculum, Marquette University, Milwaukee, Wisconsin 53233

Kenneth O. St. Louis (1), Speech Pathology and Audiology, West Virginia University, Morgantown, West Virginia 26506

[1]Present address: 7346 North Port Washington Road, Milwaukee, Wisconsin 53217.

Preface

We can be heartened by the knowledge that both the science and the art of treating stutterers has improved in recent years. With carefully applied procedures, most stutterers can be treated effectively. Nevertheless, various minority subgroups of stutterers are often *not* treated effectively; they frequently become the casualties of ordinarily effective programs.

The Atypical Stutterer: Principles and Practices of Rehabilitation is unique among the works currently available on stuttering. It focuses not on the "average" stutterer but on seven different subgroups of stutterers that clinical speech–language pathologists encounter but have difficulty managing. As the reader will discover, considerable information does exist on most of these subgroups, but it is information that is typically slighted, or ignored altogether, in textbooks and courses on stuttering. The purpose of *The Atypical Stutterer* is to summarize the information and data currently available and to provide specific diagnostic and therapeutic principles and suggestions for atypical stutterers.

St. Louis' introductory chapter presents the problem of the atypical stutterer and a rationale for writing this book. Problems such as the reality of subgroups and the issue of standardized versus customized treatments are critically analyzed. Leith's chapter, entitled "Treating the Stutterer with Atypical Cultural Influences," brings into focus a number of clinical problems that the average clinician is likely to overlook, such as cultural differences regarding eye contact, being on time, and being assertive. In "The Female Stutterer," Silverman questions such time-honored concepts as the validity of the male-to-female ratio among stutterers. Her recommended approach to diagnosis and therapy with female stutterers includes a strong emphasis on interviewing and counseling techniques. Sacco discusses special problems encountered by severe stutterers. He recommends a careful, comprehensive approach to treatment, emphasizing that reducing stuttering alone is not sufficient in treating this population. Cox focuses on the subgroup of stutterers who have concomitant psychological adjustment problems. He discusses the kind of associated psychological problems most likely to co-occur with stuttering and their roles in such issues as resistance to therapy and generalization of new speaking skills. Cooper's chapter on the mentally retarded stutterer draws together the pertinent, but rather meager, research on the topic. He recommends consideration of cognitive–attitudinal variables as well as stuttering behaviors in both diagnosis and therapy. Daly's chapter on the clutterer contains a comprehensive review of the syndrome of cluttering. He recommends a diagnostic evaluation to isolate potential associated symptoms that differentiate cluttering from stuttering components. Specific suggestions for therapy are also provided. Helm-Estabrooks, in her chapter entitled "Diagnosis and Management of Neurogenic Stuttering in Adults," carefully reviews the literature on stuttering secondary to brain damage. She develops different profiles of neurogenic stutterers depending on the nature and location of their brain damage. Specific therapeutic suggestions are provided.

This book is written primarily for clinicians who treat stutterers. Practicing speech–language pathologists and graduate student clinicians will find a wealth of insights and practical suggestions that can immediately be put to use in therapy. The book will be useful to other professional groups as well. Instructors of courses in stuttering will find well-documented reviews of the literature on most atypical categories, and researchers in the area of stuttering will discover that they are earnestly challenged to begin to include atypical subgroups in their research investigations. Professionals, such as special educators, sociologists, psychologists, nurses, aphasiologists, and teachers in women's studies, will find specific chapters of The Atypical Stutterer pertinent to their work. Each chapter includes definition(s) of the atypical category in question, pertinent literature bearing on that subgroup, diagnostic considerations, and therapeutic suggestions. Most chapters are supplemented by case studies that serve to personalize and to illustrate the need to consider separately each atypical category.

The Problem of the Atypical Stutterer: An Introduction

Kenneth O. St. Louis

PURPOSE

This book is written for persons who are engaged in the noble enterprise of understanding stutterers and helping them to improve their speech. It is not, however, like any of the books currently available that relate to the treatment of stuttering. Instead, this volume is designed to focus attention on those individuals who do not fit our conception of the "average" or "typical" stutterer. Consider the following cases:

Case 1. J. was a 26-year-old graduate student from Kenya, Africa, who manifested a mild to moderate stuttering problem. His symptoms consisted primarily of sound and word repetitions accompanied by such accessory behaviors as lip tremors, visible neck tension, and lack of eye contact. The case history revealed intermittent stuttering in his native language, beginning at about age 10, but the problem appeared to have declined over the years. J. had relatives who stuttered as well.

J. reported that at the time of the evaluation, his stuttering was limited primarily to English, which he spoke quite well

1

with a British accent. At that point, he apparently stuttered very little in his native language.

J. was not unusually fearful of his stuttering but was adamant that no one from his country find out that he was in speech therapy. Apparently, he was a chief in his native tribe, and any knowledge about his speech therapy that might get back to the tribe would seriously jeopardize his position and status at home. J. was extremely reluctant to engage in any transfer activities outside the clinic.

Case 2. W. was a 36-year-old former shipping clerk, married, with a family, when he fell and struck his head. He could neither recall the accident nor any events for several days following. His wife recalled that he had "trouble getting his words out" but that he was not "stuttering." One month later, he did begin to "stutter" and, shortly thereafter, had a "nervous breakdown." About 9 months later, he "lost his voice" and remained aphonic for another 7 months. Apparently, he had become aphonic once some years before the accident. With speech therapy, W. regained his voice but began to stutter again. Subsequent therapy for the stuttering was initially highly effective, but W. soon relapsed such that his stuttering was worse than ever.

Later, upon reevaluation at another clinic, W. stuttered on 94–100% of the words in "automatic" speech, oral reading, and conversation. He even stuttered on 90% of the words while singing "Happy Birthday." W.'s stutterings typically consisted of multiple repetitions of part of each syllable. There were associated eye blinks and mouth twitches but no evidence of avoidance.

W. also had a lateral head tremor and severe headaches emanating from the back of his neck (occipital neuralgia), which necessitated "nerve blocks" at a pain clinic. Occasionally, he had difficulty swallowing, resulting in long-term weight loss. W. was also under psychiatric care for anxiety, depression, and sexual problems. All of the other professionals treating him recommended continued speech therapy for his severe stuttering.

These cases illustrate clearly a dilemma faced by those who seek to alleviate problems of stuttering or to understand stuttering in the laboratory. There are far too many individuals who are considered to be stutterers by themselves or others who simply do not fit well into the limits of variability typically thought of as characteristic of stutterers (Rentschler, 1984). We know, for example, that most stutterers are males; are not markedly abnormal with respect to prenatal variables, motor or language development, health, personality, or intelligence; have sound/syllable repetitions and/or prolongations as their primary symptoms; and are quite likely to have accessory behaviors or "tricks" that are perceived to help them when they stutter or anticipate doing so (Andrews et al., 1983; Bloodstein, 1981; Conture, 1982). Our textbooks and courses in stuttering focus heavily, and certainly in many cases, exclusively, on the typical stutterer. Where, then, does this situation leave the clinician when he[1] must evaluate or treat an atypical stutterer, such as the two just described? The clinician is often left to temper, to modify, to ignore, or to manufacture expectations and facts to account for the unusual client he sees.

Let us hasten to add that there is absolutely nothing wrong with the clinician expanding his expectations and knowledge; quite the contrary, this is precisely what the dedicated clinician must do. Nevertheless, we believe that the clinician should have assistance in systematizing his search. Our purpose is to draw together information on atypical stutterers that is, for good reason, usually ignored in stuttering courses and covered only in cursory fashion in some textbooks. We believe that such information ought to be considered if the understanding and treatment of stuttering are to be the best they can be.

SOME TROUBLESOME ISSUES

Which Stutterers Are Atypical?

Truth, it is said, is rarely simple. And, as areas of inquiry go, stuttering must certainly rank high on the list of disciplines about which there is a great deal of confusing, contradictory information. Consideration of the atypical stutterer is not likely to clear much of the confusion surrounding stuttering and is, no doubt, going to complicate things further for those who seek simplistic understandings. Yet, the indisputable fact for all persons who have known more than two or three stutterers, regardless of their theoretical views of causation and other issues, is that all stutterers are different. Stutterers, because they are unique human beings, are, in a sense, atypical.

---

[1]For purposes of simplicity and directness, most third person pronouns referring to clinicians, clients, and others are written singly in the masculine.

How, then, can we argue that certain stutterers are sufficiently more atypical than others to warrant a chapter in this book? Perhaps such a question, which is likely to be posed, defies a logical answer; however, following is an attempt to provide a reasonable justification. As clinicians, we rely on measures of central tendency and common impressions in our understanding of the ordinary stutterer. It seems intuitively obvious that we can do the same for various categories of atypical stutterers as well. It follows, then, that we can consider those subgroups that constitute obvious and uncontested minorities (e.g., female stutterers), those that we know to exist and can easily imagine to exist in sufficient numbers to warrant a subgroup (e.g., psychologically maladjusted stutterers), and those that are reasonably well documented in the literature (e.g., clutterers). The subgroups of stutterers selected by these criteria for inclusion in this volume are those who "atypicality" results from cultural influences, gender (i.e., female), severity, psychological adjustment, cognitive ability, symptom complex (i.e., cluttering), and known neurogenic etiology.

Why Subgroup?

Another thorny issue raised in this approach is that of subgroups of stutterers in general. The notion that stuttering is not a unitary disorder has a long history, and attempts to categorize stutterers into subgroups based on etiology, symptoms, or other criteria are legion (Conture & Schwartz, 1984; Preus, 1981; Prins & Lohr, 1972; Riley & Riley, 1980; St. Onge, 1963). Van Riper (1982) reviewed a number of such attempts to subgroup stutterers over the years and concluded that the successful results to date are too disparate and too much limited to one or two factors studied for us to conclude that reliable subgroups have been identified. It is interesting to note here that Van Riper did not refer to his own developmental "tracks" as subgroups, which he described 11 years earlier (Van Riper, 1971) and left virtually unchanged in the revised edition of his book. This categorization, however imperfect, has tentatively been accepted by many in recent years and has limited empirical support (Daly, 1981; Daly & Smith, 1976, 1979; Preus, 1981). Schwartz, Conture, and Gleason (1982) proposed another typology for child stutterers for which they have considerable physiological support. Whether or not their subgroups become widely accepted remains to be seen.

The remaining chapters of this book do focus on specific subgroups of stutterers, but the subgrouping criteria and rationale are different from the attempts referred to in the above paragraph and others like them. Those endeavors ordinarily had the purpose of dividing all, or nearly all, stutterers into neat, mutually exclusive subgroups. We have no such intention. The groups represented here are meant to be neither mutually exclusive nor exhaustive. In fact, it is quite possible that a given stutterer could be considered in several of the subgroups. Additionally, clinicians will likely identify other subgroups of stutterers that reflect sufficiently unique problems to be studied and, perhaps, considered differently for remediation. Basically, the subgroups described here should be considered as a first step in identifying those minority groups of stutterers that require special consideration in conceptualization, diagnosis, and therapy.

Standardized versus Customized Therapy?

How does consideration of specific subgroups of stutterers impact upon the issue of standardized versus customized approaches to therapy for stutterers? With few exceptions, the well-known centers for stuttering therapy provide the same general approaches to practically all stutterers going through the programs. Webster (1974) argued that the Precision Fluency Shaping Program can be viewed as a standard treatment for stuttering. Ryan (1974, 1981) has developed several approaches to treating stutterers, all with the same basic therapeutic outline: establishment, transfer, and maintenance. Although establishment programs differ, Ryan does not advocate a prescriptive strategy that would target certain clients to certain treatments (Ryan & Van Kirk Ryan, 1983). Ingham (1984) has developed a standard approach to stuttering therapy using prolonged speech. He further reports that prolonged speech is the treatment which, with adult stutterers, is currently most popular and—in much of Australia, at least—perhaps has become the sole treatment taught to new clinicians.

These three examples illustrate that clinical treatment of stutterers has evolved to the point that many of the best-known clinicians in stuttering believe that standardized treatments can, and perhaps ought to be, applied to all stutterers. There is good reason for this belief (though not all authorities agree, e.g., Adams, 1982). Empirical advances in the treatment of the disorder, which have come primarily from centers such as those cited, have fortunately moved us forward from the theory-bound, "gut feeling" approaches that characterized popular approaches to stuttering therapy for many, many years (Ingham, 1984; Webster, 1977).

But the atypical stutterer remains. Is there an acceptable logic for "back-peddling" to the hazy areas of individual differences and individual treatments for stutterers with atypical situations, without denying the reality that most stutterers probably can be treated with standardized treatments? We believe there is. The chapters herein on such groups as the female stutterer, the stutterer with cluttering symptoms, or the stutterer with significant psychological maladjustment, definitely do not constitute a retreat from the empirical consensus that has served as the primary yardstick for evaluating stuttering therapies since the early 1970s (Andrews, Guitar, & Howie, 1980). Indeed, the reader will immediately recognize that several of the authors recommend existing programs for special populations that were developed with the "average" stutterer in mind. Other authors suggest adapting existing programs for the particular stratum of stutterers about which they write. It is fair to say that the overarching perspective of this volume, subscribed to in greater or lesser degree by each author, is as follows: Whenever possible, consistent, predictable, data-based treatments should be applied to all stutterers, but sensible variations should be applied to individual stutterers as needed, and, it is hoped, *before* they become the oft-ignored, small, but ever-present failure statistics (e.g., see Ingham, 1984, p. 434).

An argument could be made that, perhaps, one important difference between the master clinician and the master researcher, in spite of the continuing rhetoric by leaders in our field that they are one and the same, is their response to clinical failures. On one hand, the *clinician* knows research methodology and utilizes it diligently in his therapy, but he deviates from prescribed treatments for specific clients when it becomes clear they are about to become casualties. In this case, the research gets "clinical, " "messy," and difficult to publish. On the other hand, the *researcher* recognizes clinical processes and can perceive likely failures among his research clients, but he resists making any procedural changes that will bias the results. Here, we have solid empirical results but at the expense of a few unfortunate subjects. A case can be made that we need both the cautiously flexible clinician and the uncompromising researcher. What good are our data regarding stuttering treatments if procedures were applied in a haphazard, inconsistent fashion? And what good are standard treatments to those stutterers who, by virtue of their being atypical, cannot be reasonably expected to succeed in treatment in the usual way? There is no reason why well-informed students of stuttering could not, at different times, play one or the other of these roles.

Clearly, however, the authors in this volume are taking the side of the clinician, specifically as it relates to the problem of the atypical stutterer. The intent is to provide the clinician with additional information, insight, and suggestions to do what he does anyway, namely, to provide the best and most informed diagnostic and remedial services available.

REFERENCES

Adams, M. R. (1982). Fluency, nonfluency, and stuttering in children. *Journal of Fluency Disorders, 7,* 171–185.

Andrews, G., Craig, A., Feyer, A. M., Hoddinott, S., Howie, P., & Neilson, M. (1983). Stuttering: A review of research findings and theories circa 1982. *Journal of Speech and Hearing Disorders, 48,* 226–246.

Andrews, G., Guitar, B., & Howie, P. (1980). Meta-analysis of the effects of stuttering treatment. *Journal of Speech and Hearing Disorders, 45,* 287–307.

Bloodstein, O. (1981). *A handbook on stuttering* (3rd ed.). Chicago: National Easter Seal Society.

Conture, E. G. (1982). *Stuttering.* Englewood Cliffs, NJ: Prentice-Hall.

Conture, E. G., & Schwartz, H. D. (1984). Children who stutter: Diagnosis and remediation. *Communicative Disorders, 9,* 1–18.

Daly, D. A. (1981). Differentiation of stuttering subgroups with Van Riper's developmental tracks: A preliminary study. *Journal of the National Student Speech and Hearing Association, 9,* 89–101.

Daly, D. A., & Smith, A. (1976). *Neuropsychological differentiations in 45 "functional stutterers."* Paper presented at the Annual Convention of the American Speech and Hearing Association, Houston, TX.

Daly, D. A., & Smith, A. (1979). *Neuropsychological comparisons of "functional," "organic," and learning disabled stutterers.* Paper presented at the Annual Convention of the International Neuropsychological Society, New York, NY.

Ingham, R. J. (1984). *Stuttering and behavior therapy: Current Status and experimental foundations.* San Diego, CA: College-Hill.

Preus, A. (1981). *Attempts at identifying subgroups of stutterers.* Oslo, Norway: University of Oslo Press.

Prins, D., & Lohr, F. (1972). Behavioral dimensions of stuttered speech. *Journal of Speech and Hearing Research, 15,* 61–71.

Rentschler, G. J. (1984). Effects of subgrouping in stuttering research. *Journal of Fluency Disorders, 9,* 307–311.

Riley, G., & Riley, J. (1980). Motoric and linguistic variables among children who stutter: A factor analysis. *Journal of Speech and Hearing Disorders, 45,* 504–514.

Ryan, B. P. (1974). *Programmed therapy for stuttering in children and adults.* Springfield, IL: Thomas.

Ryan, B. P. (1981). Maintenance programs in progress—II. In E. Boberg (Ed.), *Maintenance of fluency.* (pp. 113–146). New York, Elsevier.

Ryan, B. P., & Van Kirk Ryan, B. (1983). Programmed stuttering therapy for children: Comparison of four established programs. *Journal of Fluency Disorders, 8,* 291–321.

Schwartz, H. D., Conture, E. G., & Gleason, J. R. (1982). *Subgrouping young stutterers: Preliminay observations.* Paper presented at the Annual Convention of the American Speech-Language-Hearing Association, Toronto, Ontario.

St. Onge, K. (1963). The stuttering syndrome. *Journal of Speech and Hearing Research, 6,* 195–197.

Van Riper, C. (1971). *The nature of stuttering*. Englewood Cliffs, NJ: Prentice-Hall.
Van Riper, C. (1982). *The nature of stuttering* (2nd ed.). Englewood Cliffs, NJ: Prentice-Hall.
Webster, R. L. (1974). A behavioral analysis of stuttering: Treatment and theory. In K. S. Calhoun, H. E. Adams, & K. M. Mitchell (Eds.), *Innovative treatment methods in psychopathology* (pp. 17–61). New York: Wiley.
Webster, R. L. (1977). Concept and theory in stuttering: An insufficiency of empiricism. In R. W. Rieber (Ed.), *The problem of stuttering: Theory and therapy* (pp. 65–71). New York: Elsevier.

Treating the Stutterer with Atypical Cultural Influences

William R. Leith

CULTURES IN THE UNITED STATES

We are faced with an impossible task in this chapter: to discuss all of the cultural implications present when dealing with a stuttering client whose culture differs from that of the clinician. At best, we will be able to introduce the concept of cultural influence in stuttering therapy and where it will most likely arise. The purpose of the chapter is to sensitize the reader to cultural differences and how they might influence the treatment program.

In this chapter we consider the term *culture* in its broadest interpretation: the attitudes, beliefs, behaviors, and life style of a group of people. It is the commonality of these factors among the group members that make the group homogeneous and, hence, a cutural group. Herskovits (1955) sets forth the following theoretic postulates concerning the nature of cultures: ''(1) Culture is universal in man's experience, yet each local or regional manifestation of it is unique; (2) culture is stable, yet is also dynamic, and manifests constant change; and (3) culture fills and largely determines the course of our lives, yet rarely intrudes into conscious thought'' (p. 306). Leininger (1970) writes that ''culture may be viewed as a blueprint for living which guides a particular group's thoughts, actions, and sentiments'' (p. 49). The culture of a group

9

of people is developmental in nature and is passed on from one generation to the next. Over time, cultures change in subtle ways but, in the main, the basic themes of the cultures remain relatively intact.

There seems to be a natural tendency for people to view a cultural group as an entity within itself rather than as being made up of a number of related subgroups. For example, we refer to the Hispanic culture as though it is an entity in itself. However, if we carefully examine this culture we will find subcultural groups within it. The four most obvious subcultural Hispanic groups in the United States are those groups whose cultural roots are to be found in Mexico, Latin America, the Caribbean, or Spain. These groups do indeed belong in the Hispanic culture, but their individual cultures are each distinct enough that they form separate subcultures.

Moreover, if we further examine the Caribbean Hispanic culture in the United States, we would find additional subcultural divisions. The Caribbean Hispanic culture found in the Miami area differs substantially from that found in New York City. Considering these factors, we must then view each general culture as being made up of a variety of subcultural groups and even these groups being further subdivided into unique cultural groups.

If we were to attempt to describe what would be the general culture of our nation, we would have to take the most predominant one since, as a nation settled by immigrants, innumerable cultures are represented. For the purposes of this chapter we address this culture as the *General American* culture. As with all other cultures, it developed over time, continues to change, and is made up of many subcultures.

Leavitt (1974), in studying the prevalence of stuttering in Puerto Rico and the Puerto Rican population in New York City, presents four factors which interacted to form the General American culture. The first factor concerns who the original immigrants were and where they emigrated from. The original immigrants to the United States were from Europe, and they brought with them their pride in personal achievement, a common trait in the various cultures in Europe.

The second factor was the influence of Puritanism. Leavitt (1974) states that this "denotes the theological, ethical, social, and political philosophy and way of life typical of certain Protestant groups." She goes on to say, "The development of Puritanism near the end of the sixteenth century reflected the increasing importance of the goal of individual achievement." Leavitt concludes that the influence of the Puritans included "the values of individual responsibility and initiative; thrift, diligence, and sobriety; work as an end in itself, and ceaseless activity;

success as a reward for striving, and failure as a measure of personal inadequacy; orientation to the future; utilitarianism, traditionalism, empiricism, and pragmatism; respect for science; a sense of mission; conformity, and resistance to authority" (p. 109).

The third major influence was the western frontier. It not only weakened the patriarchal family, traditional of the European and Puritan influences, it also promoted a feeling of nationalism, a sense of belonging to a unique nation. The westward movement added strength to the Puritan ethic of individualism since the frontier demanded that the pioneers be self-reliant.

The final influence was that of child rearing. Stemming from Puritanism and the influence of the frontier, children were reared to be competitive, aggressive, striving, and achievement oriented, which, as is noted later in the chapter, are factors common among cultures that are prone to have a higher incidence of stuttering. The role model provided for the children was one of independence, self-reliance, and individualism. It was the interaction of these factors that formed the core of the General American culture, namely, the Anglo–Saxon Protestant core.

Even as the General American culture was developing, immigration to the United States continued. New immigrants tended to settle in areas where earlier immigrants from their particular cultural group had already settled. In this way, cultures were maintained and passed on to future generations. However, from the earliest colonial times, a theme of "Anglo-conformity" (Gordon, 1964) was present. Americans who belonged to the Anglo-Saxon Protestant culture demanded "the complete renunciation of the immigrant's ancestral culture in favor of the behavior and values of the Angle-Saxon core group" (Gordon, 1964, p. 85). Anglo-conformity was, and still is, expected of members of other cultural groups. The theme of Anglo-conformity was present in a statement by John Quincy Adams who, in 1818, was quoted as saying, "If they (immigrants) cannot accommodate themselves to the character, moral, political and physical, of this country with all its compensating balances of good and evil, the Atlantic is always open to them to return to the land of their nativity" (Gordon, 1964, p. 94).

The United States, rich in cultural variations, was established by immigrants, and immigration has continued since its inception. Some of the major cultural groups found in our country today are the Afro-American, Hispanic, Jewish, American Indian (including the Alaskan tribes), Oriental, and Arabic cultures. However, as was pointed out earlier, each of these general cultural groups is made up of numerous subcultural groupings. Further, individuals, family groups, neighborhoods, and even communities that are associated with a particular subgroup also vary in terms of how closely they adhere to their culture's standards. There are important factors that influence this. It is these factors that negate stereotyping, the viewing of all persons who appear to belong to a cultural group as possessing all of the attitudes, beliefs, behaviors, and life style attributed to the general group. This would include such erroneous generalizations as all blacks have athletic ability, all Hispanics eat highly spiced foods, all American Indians are alcoholics, and so forth.

One factor that influences the degree to which an individual (or family) adheres to general cultural values is the degree of assimilation into the General American culture that has taken place. Although an individual may appear, because of race, religion, language, or some other factor, to belong to a particular cultural group, the individual may have adopted partially or totally the cultural values associated with the General American culture. The educational level of the individual and his or her socioeconomic level are also factors that influence the individual's attitudes, beliefs, behaviors, and life style. There is also the type of —and importance of—religion in the individual's life. All of these factors, and other more subtle ones, militate against stereotyping by cultural group.

DEVELOPMENT OF STUTTERING: CULTURAL INFLUENCES

Before we begin our discussion of stuttering and the influence of the individual's culture, it is important for us to recognize that, although much of the professional literature approaches the phenomenon of stuttering as though stutterers are a homogeneous group, the population should be viewed as heterogeneous. Of the multitude of factors associated with the phenomenon, the only two behaviors shared by all persons who stutter are repetitions and prolongations. With the exception of these two behaviors, each stutterer develops his or her unique form of stuttering and cognitive set. One of the most important influences in the development of the stutterer's individualistic form of stuttering and cognitive set is his or her culture. Thus, a major factor that militates against the view of homogeneity within the population of persons who stutter is the wide variety of cultural backgrounds to be found within the group.

Although it is not the primary purpose of this chapter to deal with cultural factors as they relate to the prevalence or incidence of stuttering, the cultural influence is worthy of note prior to our discussion of the treatment of stuttering. Rather than review the various reports and articles in this chapter, the reader is referred to the reviews by Bloodstein (1975) and Van Riper (1982). For our purposes, we consider those cultural factors that appear to contribute to a higher incidence of stuttering. The sociocultural variables we must consider when appraising cultural influences would be the cultural value placed on such attributes as competitiveness and achievement, child-rearing practices as related to the amount of pressure put on the child, attitudes toward language and expressive behaviors, and the treatment of defective or handicapped individuals in the culture.

Cultures that have all or most of these characteristics have a higher incidence of stuttering, since they are "stress cultures" or "tough" cultures. Cultures that have few if any of these characteristics have a lower incidence of stuttering, since they are not "stress cultures"; they are "easy" cultures. In discussing stressful cultures, Arsenian and Arsenian (1948) state:

> Psychological tension depends upon and varies with the properties of paths as means of reducing tension; and where a culture's paths make for easy tension-reduction in its members the culture is easy. Conversely, where a culture's paths make for difficult tension-reduction the culture is tough. (p. 379).

Leavitt (1974) contrasts a variety of sociocultural variables of easy cultures that are associated with very low incidence of stuttering with tough cultures having high incidence of stuttering. Those variables which are of primary importance in this chapter are those dealing with valued attributes, child rearing practices, speech attitudes, and cultural stress.

The easy cultures studied were those of the Ute tribe of North America, the Hausa tribe of West Africa, and the Scottish Hebrides. Within these cultures the valued attributes center around cooperation, generosity, deference to elders, industriousness, hospitality, humor, and, for the tribes, oratorical ability. The valued attributes in the tough cultures—the Kwakjutl tribe of North America, the Ibo tribe of West Africa, and the Japanese—focus on competitiveness, aggressiveness, achievement, ego strength, and, again for the tribes, oratorical ability.

The child-rearing practices of the easy cultures include child indulgence and love, joking aggression by children toward adults, and lack of physical punishment. The tough cultures' child-rearing practices differ in that they include early introduction to competitiveness, physical punishment, and emphasis on educational achievement.

The speech attitudes of the cultures also differ. In the easy cultures deliberate speech is admired, linguistic variations in younger children

are tolerated, children learn to speak at their own pace, speech is un-
hurried, and oratorical ability admired. In the tough cultures oratorical
ability is important before adolescence and is a means to achievement
and shaming rivals, the family is shamed if a child's speech is deviant,
and stuttering is often ridiculed and is a great social handicap.

Cultural stress in the easy cultures centers around fear of the authority
of the elders, superstitions, factors related to male–female roles and
marriage, and strains of close family and community relations. In the
tough cultures the main stress themes are achievement, striving, pres-
tige, fear of ridicule, repression of feelings, and intolerance of handicaps.

This concept of easy or tough cultures and cultural stress as related
to the incidence of stuttering formed the base of the research by Bullen
(1945), Johnson (1944), and Snidecor (1947). These researchers studied
the incidence of stuttering within various American Indian tribes and
reported either no stuttering incidence or a very low incidence based on
the absence of cultural pressure. Naroll (1959) stated that the incidence
of stuttering might well constitute an "index of cultural stress" for any
given culture.

Thus, as we examine the influence of the culture on the stuttering
treatment program, we must take a broad view of the culture, considering many aspects which might interfere with treatment. Again, however, it is imperative that we consider the individual and his or her family
unit as an entity within itself and not stereotype them within what would
appear to be their general cultural group.

As we consider these cultural influences, we must recognize that the
very factors that influenced the development and maintenance of the
stuttering may also influence the treatment. Therefore, we briefly discuss some of the more cogent points.

Child-Rearing Practices

There are many cultural variations of child-rearing practices, and many
of these are related to the family structure and orientation. The family
interactions in and of themselves may be instrumental in the development and maintenance of stuttering. Perhaps the most significant factor
concerns the orientation of the family toward the role of the child within
the family unit. We would be most concerned about those family units
that are oriented toward adult needs and values, a nonchild orientation.
In these family units, the child is expected to be silent, to not speak until
spoken to. Vertical communication in the family unit between the adult

members and the children is only initiated by adults, and children are directly discouraged from speaking when not spoken to. This places a great deal of stress on upward communication when the child feels he or she must communicate with an adult when not requested to do so. The child is often rebuked when such communication is initiated, regardless of the importance of what the child is attempting to communicate. This type of communication environment places a great deal of stress on all forms of communication between the child and adults. When the child speaks, he or she is intruding in an adult world and may be severely chastised for the intrusion.

The content of the vertical communication between the adults and the child is also a factor to consider. In many cultures the vertical communication from an adult to a child is almost always in the form of a command, instructions, or a reprimand. There is no dialogue or conversation involved, and if the child is requested to respond, the response must be as short as possible, usually limited to "yes" and "no" responses. Here, again, we find that verbal communication is a stressful activity.

Another factor that might well contribute to the development or maintenance of stuttering would be that of expectations of the family unit for achievement by the children. This family unit may be either adult or child oriented, but the parents have high expectations of the child in a variety of activities including, in some cultures, speech performance. The child is placed under a great deal of pressure to perform, and if he fails to live up to the expectations, he is penalized.

Reactions to Stuttering

The reactions to the child's stuttering by adults, peers, and other children will, for the most part, depend on the cultural beliefs about the cause of stuttering. The cultural group may believe that stuttering is due to some religious or superstitious factor such as the child being "possessed" or "under the evil eye." The evil eye is a common belief among the majority of the world's cultures and is discussed in greater detail later in the chapter. With religious or superstitious overtones, the reactions to the child and the stuttering will be essentially negative in nature, and the child would be made aware of his being possessed or under the evil eye. This may be a source of great shame for the family, and the members would react accordingly. It would not be unusual for the child to be subjected to a variety of religious or superstitious "treatments" such as special ritualistic dances, prayers, and folk remedies.

Other cultures, not having this foreboding view of the origins of stuttering, might react with open ridicule, feeling that the stuttering child is foolish. Another reaction might be anger based on the belief that the child is stuttering on purpose. However, with either reaction, the child who stutters might well be rejected by members of his or her cultural group.

The reactions to stuttering found among the various cultural groups may not differ significantly from those found in the General American culture. However, they are more pervasive, involving the entire cultural community, as opposed to the more individualistic negative reations found in the General American culture. Stutterers are thus exposed to two classes of responses to their stuttering, the predictable one from their cultural group and the unpredictable reactions they receive from persons from other cultures, including the General American culture.

In a more general view of reactions toward stuttering, we must consider the family orientation in terms of patriarchal or matriarchal societies. If the society is patriarchal, that is, the male is the dominant force in the family unit, stuttering in the male child is considered a most serious problem, since it will influence his role in the society. In that the female is subservient to the male, the seriousness of her stuttering problem is more related to her marriageability than to her place in the society. The stuttering problem in the female will be viewed more seriously in the matriarchal society, since the female role in the society is more important. The stuttering now influences not only the female child's marriageability but also her future role in the society.

Special Clinical Factors

All speech clinicians who work with clients who stutter will come in contact with clients and their significant others who are influenced by cultures other than that of the clinician. The type and degree of influence depends primarily on what particular cultural group or subgroup the client is associated with, the degree of assimilation into the General American Culture, the educational level, the socioeconomic level, and so forth. In that there are an infinite number of variations within each general cultural group, we are not able to discuss specific cultural groups, since this would lead to stereotyping, the very thing we are trying to avoid. We can only point out possible problem areas in working with stutterers and/or significant others who might be influenced by cultural factors.

As we discuss cultural influences in stuttering treatment, there are two cultural variations that are paramount for the clinician, the first being the role that speech plays in the particular culture. As we discuss this, keep in mind that we are not making a generalization of this feature, only saying that it is a theme often found in a particular culture. There are cultures, such as some American Indian cultures, where silence is important. Members of these cultures speak only when there is something of importance to say. Compared to the General American culture, members of these cultures may appear to be nonverbal. Conversely, there are other cultures, such as some subcultural groups of the Afro-American culture, where skillful use of speech is an important source of recognition and power (Leith and Mims, 1975). Morgenstern (1953), investigating the incidence of stuttering in various cultures, reported a high incidence of stuttering in the Ibo and Idoma groups of West Africa. In addition to these cultures being competitive, achievement oriented, and emphasizing education, he reported that verbal facility was greatly admired and fluency failures were strongly ridiculed. Members of these cultures often engage in verbal games to demonstrate their skill. So, depending on the cultural influence, the importance of speech varies from being a relatively unimportant aspect of life within the cultural community to a major source of community recognition. This cultural view of speech can have a direct impact not only on the development of stuttering but also on the treatment of the disorder.

The second cultural factor that will have a direct impact on the treatment of stuttering is related to the role of the male in a particular culture. There are cultures where the male role includes the valued attribute of strength, both physical and mental. In the Japanese culture, the male can "lose face" by admitting to or yielding to fear. The cultural male role in many Mediterranean countries includes what is commonly referred to as *machismo*, or acting *macho*. The cognitive set of this macho male role model can prove to be detrimental to therapy in that the male stutterer has great difficulty admitting to and dealing with his fear of stuttering. He feels that admitting his fear or allowing others to see his stuttering, as expected in some treatment programs, is a sign of weakness. He may also experience great difficulty in dealing with this aspect of his stuttering with a female clinician. This is, of course, dependent on his cultural view of the female. If, in his culture, the female is subservient to the male, the clinical relationship may be tenuous at best. This relationship is discussed in greater detail later in the chapter.

As we conclude this section, we can draw some general conclusions regarding the role of culture in the development of stuttering. Those cultures that have a high incidence of stuttering have common characteristics that make them stressful or tough cultures. Stuttering would appear to be related to the anxiety, fear, and frustration common in tough cultures, with the children of these cultures reacting negatively to stresses as they attempt to meet cultural demands. One relatively common reaction would appear to be the development of stuttering. Any cultural group in the United States that possesses these characteristics— a tough culture—would, in all likelihood, have a higher incidence of stuttering than an easy culture. Again, it is important to note that the cultural characteristics that precipitated the stuttering may also be influencing the stutterer when he or she enters a treatment program. The clinician must be aware of these influences if they are negatively affecting the treatment process.

TREATMENT OF STUTTERING: CULTURAL INFLUENCES

The clinician faces the influence of many cultural factors in her clinical contacts with stutterers. This is not a rare instance. All persons have a cultural base and, most often, this base differs in subtle ways from that of the clinician. In many instances the differences are not significant enough to create problems in therapy, but the factors are still operating. We are primarily concerned here with cultural differences that interfere with the clinical process. We must also recognize that clinicians who themselves are not of the General American culture face cultural influences they might not understand as they work with stutterers from that culture. The task of dealing with cultural influences faces all clinicians, regardless of their own cultural orientation.

Due to the number of factors unique to each cultural group and its related subgroups, it is impossible to discuss the influences of any specific group. Rather, we consider various aspects of the treatment process and discuss possible cultural factors that might interfere with the clinical process. Obviously, we cannot consider all cultural influences. Those that are discussed below are some of the more obvious ones. In the following discussion, a clinical example is given and then the cultural factor discussed in broader terms. In some of the discussions, possible solutions are presented, but in others, there are no obvious solutions. The clinician must work around the problems to the best of her ability, recognizing that the negative influences may be beyond her control.

Pretherapy Evaluation

Time Factors

Example. The agency has contacted a family and made an appointment for 10:00 for the evaluation of their child's stuttering. The family does not arrive at the agency until 10:30, and the clinician is upset about their late arrival, since she has another evaluation scheduled for 11:00. She openly displays her displeasure, mentioning several times that they were late for their appointment. She takes the family to the clinic room and immediately begins to ask questions about the child's developmental history. Because of the late arrival of the family, the evaluation cannot be completed that day so another evaluation is scheduled for the following week. The family is late again, and the clinician "lectures" the parents about being on time. Since she is again running late, she starts to work on the evaluation as soon as the family is in the clinic room. The parents are uncooperative during the evaluation, and when the evaluation is completed and a recommendation is made for the child to receive therapy, the parents reject the recommendation.

Discussion. The clinician was dealing with a family whose culture is not time oriented. These cultures do not feel the pressure to be on time that is common in the clinician's culture. There are many cultures that are not time oriented, perhaps the most common of which is the American Indian culture. If this is the family's orientation to the time factor, the clinician must recognize it and adjust for it if the child is to receive therapy.

The second cultural factor the clinician faced was that of beginning to discuss "business" before taking the time for social interaction. This is considered impolite by many cultures. Regardless of the time factor, the clinician should have taken the time for some general social interactions with the family (rapport, if you will) before she began her history taking and the acual evaluation. Failure to take time for these social amenities may alienate the family to the point where an evaluation is impossible.

Who Speaks for the Family

Example. In taking a child's developmental history, the clinician addresses her questions to the mother, assuming that the mother would be the one who would have the information. The clinician is frustrated and confused because the mother remains silent while the father attempts to answer the questions. It is obvious that the father does not have the needed information so the clinician becomes more obvious in directing the questions to the mother. She finally asks the father if he will allow the mother to answer the question. He becomes silent and rather sullen but remains silent. However, regardless of the question directed to her, the mother remains silent. The evaluation cannot be completed so the clinician attempts to schedule another meeting with the family. The father refuses to bring the child back, and all clinical contacts with the family are lost.

Discussion. In this family's culture, the husband speaks for the family, and the wife never speaks when the husband is present. When the clinician insisted that the mother respond to the questions, she was breaking two cultural demands: that the husband speak for the family and that the wife never speak when the husband is present. She might have been able to adjust for this factor by having another clinician interview the father in one room while she spoke to the mother in another room.

While some cultures expect the husband to be the spokesperson for the family while the wife remains silent, other cultures allow the wife to be involved in a conversation while the husband is present. The best way to adjust for this factor is to address the questions generally to both parents and let them decide who will respond. If the husband is the only one who responds, while the wife remains silent, the clinician should attempt to separate them and see if, with this arrangement, the wife will respond and answer the questions.

In this situation the clinician is dealing with a culture where the father is the "law." He is not challenged in his decisions that affect the family. The clinician must deal with the father in such a way that he does not feel challenged and that, if the decision is made that the child may receive therapy, he made the decision. If the clinician is demanding or "pushy," the father will reject her and her suggestions. In this situation the clinician should take extreme care not to insinuate that the father contributed in any way to the child's stuttering. This would be the ultimate insult.

Female Role

Example. In interviewing the family, the clinician finds that the father speaks for the family while the mother remains silent. As she progresses with the interview, the father becomes agitated and hostile. He refuses to answer some questions and answers others with very short answers that do not provide the requested information. As the clinician persists in her questioning, the father becomes upset to the point where he leaves the interview room with the mother, and the evaluation is at an end.

Discussion. The clinician is confronted with two aspects of the cultural male and female roles. First, in this family's culture, the female is subservient to the male, never speaking in his presence and never questioning him. The father is now confronted with a female who does not fit into the cultural role model. Not only is the female clinician speaking directly to him, she is asking him questions and, on some occasions, questioning his answers. Second, the situation is compounded by the female being a figure of authority. Females in his culture do not assume an authority role, and the father cannot deal with a female in what should be, culturally, a male role. This is both insulting and threatening.

Asking about Family Matters

Example.   As part of the evaluation, the clinician wants to determine family interactions and responses to the child and his stuttering. She asks about the relationships between the family members. The parents become more and more uneasy and guarded in their responses. Their answers are vague and not in direct response to the questions. In her frustration, the clinician becomes more demanding and more personal in her questions. The parents become very upset and walk out of the interview. They leave the agency with their child and do not make any further contacts for an evaluation.

Discussion.   Within this family's culture, family matters are private and not to be shared with strangers. The clinician insulted the family by invading their privacy. In this instance, the clinician will have to plan therapy based on the general information she can get from the family and not demand more detailed information. The lack of information may have some detrimental effect on the efficiency of her therapy, but it will not prevent therapy from being applied.

Parent's Beliefs

Example.   During the evaluation of a young stutterer, the clinician tells the mother what a nice child she has, how polite and well behaved he is. She continues to praise the mother periodically during the evalua-tion. Each time the clinician praises the child, the mother becomes more uneasy and agitated. The clinician, seeing the mother's uneasiness, feels that the mother is reacting this way because of her embarrassment about the stuttering. In order to counteract this, the clinician praises the child even more. The mother becomes more agitated with each instance of praise and finally takes the child out of the clinic room and leaves the agency. Repeated attempts to get the child back for an evaluation fail.

Discussion.   The clinician inadvertently caused the mother to think that she was going to abduct or "possess" the child. The mother felt that the clinician was casting a spell on the child with the evil eye. This particular belief, the evil eye, is a widely held belief in the world's cul-tures, with over half of the cultures believing in some form of influence by the evil eye. Although it takes different forms, the intent remains the same. The evil eye is a source of power, with one person taking over or possessing another person. Each culture has rituals, objects, or other means of warding off the evil eye. For example, a pendent commonly worn by Italian men in the shape of a curled horn is to ward off the evil eye.

When someone is felt to be possessed by the evil eye, these same cultures have rituals to rid the person of its effects. These rituals can take the form of, for example, dances, ingesting special foods, religious ceremonies, or washing or rubbing the skin with special substances. In some cultures it is felt that stuttering is the result of the person being possessed by the evil eye.

Other beliefs are more directly related to the stuttering itself. The parents may believe that the stuttering is a sign that the child is already possessed by the evil eye or that the stuttering is a religious curse. Still others may feel that the child is stuttering on purpose or that this is an indication that the child is defective. These beliefs will have an impact on therapy, which is discussed in more detail in the section entitled "Stuttering Therapy."

Being Alone with Strangers

Example. Having met the family in the waiting room, the male clinician attempts to take the child, a 14-year-old female, to the clinic room for an evaluation of the stuttering. The father insists on accompanying the child for the evaluation. The clinician, feeling that the father would inhibit the child and negatively influence the evaluation, insists that he stay in the waiting room. The father continues to insist that he accompany his daughter, and the clinician attempts to explain why he wants to see the child alone. After a short discussion, the parents take the child and leave the agency.

Discussion. The family's culture does not allow the female child to be alone with a male stranger, that is, a male that is not related to her by family. If the child must be with a stranger, she is accompanied by a male member of her family. By insisting that the father remain in the waiting room, the clinician offered the family no recourse but to leave. They could not go against their cultural mores by allowing their daughter to be alone with a male stranger. If the clinician had been more sensitive to the issue, he would have allowed the father to accompany his daughter or see if the client could be assigned to a female clinician. Either of these actions would have resolved the problem. Many cultures are extremely protective of the female, and this can create problems in either the evaluation or the treatment of stuttering.

Touching the Client

Example. The speech clinician is evaluating the speech of a young female stutterer. The mother and the child are in the room and, after the evaluation is completed, the clinician, attempting to reward the child for her good behavior, pats her on her head. The mother becomes upset and is uncooperative during the rest of the conference. She refuses to allow the child to receive therapy.

Discussion. In this family's culture, the hair is considered sacred and not to be touched by a stranger. The clinician, in touching the hair, broke a religious rule and insulted the family. Other cultures do not allow a stranger to even see the female's hair, requiring the female to wear a head scarf that completely covers the hair.

Members of some cultures do not even allow a stranger—a person who is not related by blood—to touch them. This touching taboo may be generalized, or it may apply to a specific part of the body. To touch the face can be interpreted as extremely personal and the individual— child or adult—may be insulted if it occurs.

There is also a potential problem in some cultures if a female touches an adult male. The touching may be interpreted as aggressive or even sexual behavior. This has serious overtones, and if the clinician touches a male client, it not only can lead to an awkward situation but can destroy the client/clinician relationship.

Stuttering Therapy

The continuous and close interpersonal relationships involved in the therapy process presents additional problems in terms of cultural influences. Again, all of the potential problems cannot be foreseen, but some of the more obvious ones are discussed in this section.

Selection of Treatment Program

Example. The treatment program selected by the clinician for the 16-year-old male stutterer calls for the client to stutter openly in one phase of treatment. The client resists this phase of treatment and continually fails to do his clinical assignments of open stuttering. The clinician insists that the client perform the clinical tasks and puts pressure on the client to stutter openly outside the clinical environment. The client becomes upset with the clinical demands and withdraws from the clinical program.

Discussion. In the client's culture, fluent speech is highly regarded, while dysfluent speech is ridiculed. The clinician, in demanding that the client stutter openly, is asking the client to subject himself to ridicule by the members of his culture. The client is forced to make a choice of following either the instructions of the clinician or the dictates of his culture. Because of the negative reactions to his dysfluent speech by members of his culture, he chose to withdraw from therapy.

The clinician should have selected a fluency-oriented treatment program rather than one that included the "broadcasting" or "advertising" of the stuttering as part of the treatment. Had the clinician made this selection, he would not have forced the client to decide between the rather abstract benefits of therapy and the very real penalties he would receive from his culture.

However, even the fluency-oriented programs present some problems for the client. There are many cultures whose native language is spoken quite rapidly. Members of these cultures also speak English very rapidly, and this becomes the cultural norm in the group. If someone were to speak at a very slow rate, this would constitute abnormal speech and could also be ridiculed. Thus, if the treatment program is based on rate control, even though the client might be "fluent," the speech would still be considered abnormal by his or her cultural counterparts.

Cultures that focus on verbal facility may also react negatively to slow speech, even though it may be fluent. Slow speech does not lend itself to verbal facility: to be verbally quick, to carry on a running verbal string. Here again, we have a possible source of ridicule in the culture since verbal facility often means speaking fast. The client will be at a disadvantage in speaking with peers while using a slow rate of speech. His sociocultural need is not fluency as related to stuttering, but rather unique verbal fluency as defined by his culture (Leith and Mims, 1975).

Time Factors

Example. The adult male client is consistently late for his appointments, and this creates problems for the clinician, since clinical appointments are back to back. The clinician talks to the client about this, but there is no change in the client's behavior. Progress in therapy is being negatively affected because of the reduced amount of clinical time the clinician has with the client.

Discussion. The clinician is dealing with another facet of cultural beliefs associated with time. In this client's culture, to arrive anywhere at the appointed time is considered an insult to the other person, an insinuation that they have nothing else to do. Vestiges of this belief are found in many other cultures where people arrive at social gatherings "fashionably late." Perhaps the clinician could schedule this client to arrive for therapy 15 minutes earlier than his actual appointment time. This arrangement might reduce the amount of time the clinician must wait for him to arrive.

Gender of the Clinician

Example.   A female clinician is working with a male stutterer who is slightly older than she is. His attitude in therapy is basically negative. He is uncooperative and responds to her in a rather hostile manner. She tries to establish better rapport with him but cannot. He continues in therapy but clinical progress is very slow.

Discussion.   In this client's culture, the female is subservient to the male. Females who do not follow the cultural standard and are assertive, perhaps even aggressive, are often viewed as being immoral. The client resents the female role the clinician has assumed, and the resentment is evidenced in his hostile behavior and his lack of cooperation.

In the event that the clinician has selected a treatment program that includes working with the client's emotional involvement with the stuttering, this could create severe clinical problems. If the client's cultural male role is macho oriented, the client will have great difficulty in admitting that he is fearful of the stuttering and even greater difficulty in dealing with it. A client cannot deal with fear if he denies it exists. Even if it is presented logically—that if there were no fear of stuttering, there would be no secondary mannerisms since there is nothing fearful to avoid—the client will deny it. To add to the complexity of the clinical situation, the client is being asked to admit his fear to a female clinician, and the female is one of the main reasons that the macho image exists.

We also have a problem in this example because the clinician is younger than the client. This is also the source of resentment, the young female delving into his "weakness," his fear of stuttering. His reaction to this is one of defensiveness and anger. He cannot display his vulnerability to stuttering to a female clinician, let alone one who is younger than he is.

There may be still other factors involved in this male–female conflict situation. The resentment may stem from the male having to be taught by a younger female. Another aspect of the conflict might be the client reacting to a young female speaking to a stranger. The relationships between males and females in various cultures are complex, and the clinician should be aware of the possible conflicts that can arise in a clinical situation.

Eye Contact

Example. One of the clinical goals in the treatment program the clinician is applying is to have the client maintain eye contact with the listener. The client, a 22-year-old female, never maintains eye contact with the clinician, whether she is speaking or not. The more the clinician insists on eye contact, the more upset the client becomes. The client finally withdraws from therapy.

Discussion. The clinician failed to realize that, in the client's culture, maintaining eye contact is a sign of aggressive, or even hostile, behavior. Direct eye contact is a negative behavior in the culture, while the lowering of the eyes is a sign of respect. Further, for a female to maintain eye contact has an even more serious overtone, that of being sexually aggressive. The behavior the clinician requested of the client was not only culturally unacceptable in terms of hostile–aggressive behavior, it also would create a stigma for the client, suggesting that she was sexually aggressive.

There are many cultures where the maintaining of eye contact is a negative behavior. This creates problems for clinicians whose treatment program includes the clinical goal of having the client maintain eye contact while speaking. In the General American culture, direct eye contact is a valued social attribute. Those persons in the culture who do not maintain eye contact are often labeled "shifty eyed," which is an indication that they are not to be trusted. Lack of eye contact is associated with lying.

When direct eye contact is a clinical demand, the client is forced to make a choice between the demands of therapy and those of her culture. If she chooses therapy and maintains eye contact, her cultural counterparts will penalize the behavior, and she will acquire a negative reputation. The sociocultural costs are too great, and she must yield to the demands of her culture and withdraw from therapy. She must live in her culture and with the members of the culture. Her social position and reputation is determined by her culture and this by far outweighs the possible, but abstract, benefits of therapy.

Gestures

Example. The clinician is working with an adult female client. During a clinical session, the client is doing an outstanding job on her speech, and the clinician wants to reward her as she is speaking. In order to reward the client and not interrupt her, the clinician uses a gesture. The gesture consists of touching the tip of the thumb with the index finger, forming a circle. When the gesture is presented to the client, she stops speaking and glares at the clinician. There is a great deal of tension in the clinic room for the remainder of the session, and the client requests a different clinician.

Discussion. Although this gesture is a positive one in the clinician's culture, it is an obscenity in the client's. The client was insulted by the clinician's behavior. Also, since the clinician did not realize what she had done, she could not explain the gesture to the client. Gestures are used by all cultures to express both positive and negative messages, and the same gesture may carry different messages in different cultures. There are even some cultures that consider any gesturing with the left hand an insult.

Impolite Behavior

Example. The clinician is working with an 18-year-old female stutterer. The client is having particular difficulty with the *th* sound, having severe blocks on it. The treatment program the clinician is using calls for teaching the client a method of gaining voluntary control over the block to terminate it. In order to teach the technique to the client, the clinician models the technique. However, the client will not watch her perform the model and will not attempt to imitate it.

Discussion. The client will not watch the clinician model the behavior or attempt it herself because, in her culture, exposing the tongue is an extremely impolite behavior. In attempting to teach the behavior, the clinician exaggerated the tongue position so the client could see it clearly. This was embarrassing for the client, as was the request by the clinician for her to perform the behavior. The clinician might well approach this by modifying the *th* sound so that the tongue was barely visible between the teeth. With this type of presentation the client might be able to tolerate the model and even perform the behavior.

Transfer the New Speech

Example. The 12-year-old male client has progressed in therapy to the point where the clinician feels that the new speech behavior should be generalized to the home and other speaking environments. She gives the client assignments to use his new speech in other speaking situations. Over a period of time there is no evidence that the new speech is generalizing outside the clinical environment. The parents report that the new speech is not evident in the home. The clinician cannot get the new speech generalized.

Discussion. The family's culture is not child oriented. Children are to be seen but not heard. The client is not allowed to initiate a conversation with an adult. His verbal interactions with adults are limited to responding to questions or orders. Further, his verbal responses are expected to be as brief as possible, and the level of communication stress in this situation interferes with the production of the new speech. Thus, he has limited opportunities to use his new speech except with his peers. Generalization of the new speech will be severely limited.

If the clinician is working with a young woman whose culture does not allow her to speak to strangers, new problems of transfer of the new speech arise. Although the client may be able to use the new speech in the clinical environment, and even with her relatives, she will have very limited opportunities to use it with other people, particularly with males. In some cultures, if the young lady is in school, she will be able to speak with classmates and teachers but not outside the school environment. Still others will allow the female to speak to clerks in stores and in other business-related activities, but social verbal interaction is not allowed. All of these limitations inhibit the generalization of the new speech.

Nonverbal Client

Example. The clinician is working with a young male stutterer. She has explained carefully the new speech behaviors she wants him to use so that he will be more fluent. Therapy is now moving into a conversational mode so the client can practice using the new speech behaviors. However, no matter what the clinician does, she cannot get spontaneous, ongoing speech from the client. He will only respond to direct questions, and even then his responses are limited to one- or two-word answers.

Discussion. There are several possible reasons for this problem. The most obvious reason is that the child comes from a culture where children are not to speak unless they are spoken to. The child has never had the opportunity to converse openly with an adult. The clinician will have great difficulty in getting the child to converse with her since this is a cultural taboo. If the client was a female and the clinician was male, we would have still another problem, which was discussed earlier under the section concerning the gender of the clinician and the client. Still another possibility would be that the child, because of a lack of contact and experience, is fearful of speaking to a person of another culture.

Parents' Beliefs

Example. The client in this example is a 5-year-old male. The clinician is successful in establishing new speech in therapy. However, in each succeeding contact she has with the client, there is no carryover of the new speech behavior from the previous session. After several clinical meetings, the clinician asks the child why he is not trying to use the new speech behavior. The child responds that he is punished at home when he tries to use the new speech.

Discussion. Even though the parents agreed that the child could receive therapy, because of their cultural religion, they believe that the child's stuttering is their religious punishment for something they have done. The stuttering can be removed only if they atone for their sins, and, when this is done, the stuttering will disappear. Therapy is threatening this belief by changing the stuttering, thereby reducing their punishment. They must maintain the child's stuttering because of their religious beliefs.

Though the clinician may speak to the parents about their beliefs regarding stuttering, it does not mean that their beliefs have changed. Further, they may have even signed permission forms for the child to receive therapy. However, they may still subject the child to religious and superstitious rituals to alleviate the stuttering. If they believe that the child is stuttering on purpose, they may react with anger and punitive behavior when the stuttering occurs. The parents' reactions to the child and his stuttering will have a significant impact on the effectiveness of the therapy.

RESOURCES FOR CLINICIANS

Reference materials are an important resource for the clinician dealing with a client whose stuttering is culturally influenced; several are included in the References and Recommended Readings section of this chapter. Another source of information would be departments of anthropology at colleges and universities. Faculty members should be able to recommend readings and/or discuss the cultural group the clinician is dealing with.

If the clinician is working in a school environment where there are bilingual teachers, these teachers can serve as resources, since they deal with children from many cultures. The clinician might even turn to other professionals such as other clinicians, teachers, psychologists, and social workers whose general cultural group is the same as the particular client or who have had extensive experience with the client's particular culture.

Unfortunately, the profession of speech–language pathology has not dealt with the issue of providing services to persons whose culture is different from that of the clinician. The field of nursing is dealing with this issue with a specialty area in transcultural nursing. Since both the nurse and the speech clinician are involved in interpersonal relations with their patients or clients, we can take advantage of the advances this field has made in transcultural interpersonal relationships. The most meaningful reference for the speech clinician would be the book, *Nursing and Anthropology: Two Worlds to Blend*, by Leininger (1970). Another health-related reference the clinician will find helpful is *Health Professional/Patient Interaction*, by Purtilo (1978). Two more general books that will provide an overview of cultures and their influences on life-styles are *Cultural Anthropology*, by Herskovits, (1955) and *Naciremas*, by Spradley and Rynkiewich (1975).

In 1980, a 3-day conference on "Cultural Influences in Communication Disorders" was held at Wayne State University in Detroit, Michigan. The conference was designed to meet the needs of the speech clinicians and the bilingual teachers in the public schools. After presentations of Arabic, Afro-American, Indian, Hispanic, and Oriental cultures were made, discussions were held concerning cultural influences in the treatment of articulation and language disorders as well as stuttering. The conference participants developed a list of recommendations for speech clinicians who find themselves working with a client whose cultural background is different from their own. Those recommendations that are broad in scope as well as those directly related to the stuttering client are presented below. Some of the recommendations are discussed earlier in the chapter. The list is provided as a quick overview and reference for the reader.

Conference Recommendations

1. It is extremely important for speech clinicians to recognize that there is no standard cultural group. Each group represents a wide variety of subcultures, depending on the degree of assimilation into the

General American culture, the socioeconomic level of the subculture, the geographic location of the subculture, the educational level of the members of the subculture, and so forth. There are also individual family variations within the subculture influenced by the above-mentioned factors. Cultural orientation will only give direction to questions concerning the importance of general cultural influences. This awareness of variability will help prevent cultural stereotyping on the part of the clinician.

2. Some cultures are extremely private about their family and personal lives. The clinician should respect this privacy and not discuss such matters if the client is from such a culture.

3. Some cultures protect their children to the point where the child has great difficulty in adjusting to the school setting. This could include dealing with adults, other than family members, on a one-to-one basis.

4. Within some cultures it is impolite to speak in a "loud" voice. A child from one of these cultures might speak very softly, to the point where it is difficult to understand what is being said. This may not be shyness, but rather, a cultural influence carried over from the home.

5. Since various cultures respond to the handicapped in different ways, it is very important for the clinician to know the response of the client's culture to handicapped persons.

6. Establishing rapport with the family may be difficult if the clinician is female and the culture of the family does not accept the female in this type of role. There may also be problems if the clinician is from another culture. Both of these factors may be compounded by the fact that the clinician represents a "figure of authority."

7. The role of the child within the family unit varies from culture to culture. If the cultural family unit is child oriented, a home program may be able to be instituted, since the parents are involved with their children. However, if the cultural family unit is not child oriented, parental cooperation is not likely to occur, regardless of attempts on the part of the clinician.

8. In cultures that are not child oriented, the parents are usually not involved in the child's efforts in the school environment. It may be advisable to increase the rewards and encouragement the child receives in the school environment to compensate for the lack of support from the home.

9. In some cultures, the female rarely comes in contact with people of other cultures, relating only with people of her own culture. This can create problems both in terms of home visits by the clinician and the establishment of home programs.

10. There may be instances where a child is unwilling to communicate

with a person of another culture. The clinician should be sensitive to this possibility.

11. Failure on the part of a child to maintain eye contact with the clinician may be a cultural factor. It should not be misinterpreted as an attitudinal sign or a secondary mannerism associated with stuttering.

12. Depending on the culture, it may not be appropriate for the clinician to touch the child. This is particularly true for some Indian tribes where the hair is considered sacred. A pat on the head would be most inappropriate with a child from such a tribe.

13. If the family is required to sign forms or other documents for the testing of a child, this may, depending on the culture, embarrass or shame the family. If this is the case, the parents may not sign the forms or documents.

14. Mannerisms used by a bilingual child to cover up his or her lack of English proficiency may be misinterpreted as secondary mannerisms associated with stuttering. The clinician should check to see if the mannerisms occur when the child is speaking his or her native language. If not, there is still a possibility that the child is stuttering while speaking English. This factor should be checked very carefully and appropriate action taken if the child is stuttering.

15. If a child is demonstrating some stuttering in his or her native language, it would be advisable to remedy the stuttering problem before enrolling the child in a program for English as a second language. Communication stress is an important factor in the development and maintenance of stuttering, and the demands for learning and speaking English would create even more communication stress on the child and make the problem worse.

17. Communiative stress can often be found within the culture itself if oral ability is a source of peer recognition and status. Various cultures view oral ability as an important factor for status within the community. This cultural attitude can have a profound effect on the treatment of stuttering. The clinician should be aware of this factor and determine its influence on the particular child she is working with.

18. Various cultures have different attitudes towards stuttering, and it is important that the clinician determine the attitude of the family. In some cultures it is viewed as a curse or has some religious overtones. The family's attitude will have a direct influence on the treatment of the problem.

19. Many stuttering treatment programs stress the importance of eye contact as a goal of therapy. The clinician should keep in mind that this is considered a negative behavior in many cultures, particularly for the female.

Discussion

The viability of the profession of speech–language pathology is dependent on the efficiency and effectiveness of the clinical services it offers. This is the "product" of the profession. Without this product, the profession would have no reason to exist. Research in human communication and communication disorders serves as a foundation for the clinical services offered, providing additional information so that the effectiveness and efficiency of therapy can be improved. There is an important symbiotic relationship between the researcher and the clinician, but the relationship is dependent on communication between the parties. Researchers communicate with the clinicians through publications in professional journals. However, clinicians have limited means of communicating their needs to the researcher. This is one of the purposes of this chapter: to communicate a clinical need to the researcher.

It would seem obvious that various cultures influence both the development and the treatment of stuttering. And, it appears obvious that the clinician must take the cultural influence into consideration when selecting an appropriate treatment program and in the clinical application of that program. There are no "hard data" concerning the interactions between cultures and stuttering, but the existing empirical evidence would certainly support the thesis that they are interrelated. If clinical services to the stutterer are to be made more effective and efficient, the clinician needs more information on these interactions in order to better adjust the treatment to the individual client. This, then, represents a challenge to the researchers: to more fully investigate these interactions and make the information available to the clinicians.

Until this area is more fully researched and additional information is available, clinicians must rely on their own professional judgments and available resources. Most important of all is that they recognize that there is no "right" or "wrong," or "good" or "bad," or "pure" cultures. There are only "different" cultures.

REFERENCES AND RECOMMENDED READINGS

Arsenian, J., and Arsenian, J. (1948). Tough and easy cultures. *Psychiatry, 11,* 377–385.
Bloodstein, O. (1975). *A handbook on stuttering* (rev. ed.). Chicago: The National Easter Seal Society for Crippled Children and Adults.
Bullen, A. K. (1945). A cross-cultural approach to the problem of stuttering. *Child Development, 16,* 1–88.
Gordon, M. M. (1964). *Assimilation in American life.* New York: Oxford University Press.
Herskovits, M. J. (1955). *Cultural anthropology* (p. 306). New York: Knopf.

Johnson, W. (1944). The Indians have no word for it. *Quarterly Journal of Speech, 30,* 330–337.

Leavitt, R. R. (1974). *The Puerto Ricans: Cultural change and language deviance.* Viking Fund Publications in Anthropology, No. 51. Tucson, AZ: The University of Arizona Press.

Leininger, M. (1970). *Nursing and anthropology: Two worlds to blend.* New York: Wiley.

Leith, W. R., and Mims, H. A. (1975). Cultural influences in the development and treatment of stuttering: A preliminary report on the black stutterer. *Journal of Speech and Hearing Disorders, 40,* 459–466.

Morgenstern, J. J. (1953). *Psychological and social factors in children's stammering.* Unpublished Ph.D. dissertation, University of Edinburgh, Scotland.

Naroll, R. (1959). A tentative index of cultural stress. *International Journal of Social Psychiatry, 5,* 105–116.

Purtilo, R. (1978). *Health professional/Patient interaction.* Philadelphia: Saunders.

Snidecor, J. C. (1947). Why the Indian does not stutter. *Quarterly Journal of Speech, 33,* 493–495.

Spradley, J. P., and Rynkiewich, M. A. (1975). *Naciremas.* Boston: Little-Brown.

Van Riper, C. (1982). *The nature of stuttering* (2nd ed.). Englewood Cliffs, NJ: Prentice-Hall.

The Female Stutterer

Ellen-Marie Silverman

INTRODUCTION

There is no fact about the problem of stuttering more universally accepted than that more males than females develop the problem (Bloodstein, 1981). Wherever surveys have been conducted—in the United States, Australia, the British Isles, Europe, or South Africa—approximately four males have been identified as stutterers for each female so identified. This finding, apparently interpreted to mean that stuttering was a problem of males, probably has contributed to the scarcity of identifiable female subjects in research studies. Women either have been excluded as subjects or their responses have been pooled with those of the men studied. There are a few notable exceptions; for example, Johnson (1959, 1961) systematically studied male and female stutterers, and so did Sheehan (1979; Sheehan and Zelen, 1955), but only recently have researchers begun to routinely report male and female responses separately. As a consequence, most of what we know about stuttering and the problem of stuttering has come from the study of males, and, as such, our data base might not be entirely appropriate for theorizing

35

about the nature of stuttering, developing methods of treatment, or meeting the needs of female stutterers.

There are some data that suggest that treatment efforts based on such biased data may be unsatisfactory for females (Silverman, 1982). The data reveal that certified speech–language pathologists tend to hold negative stereotypes of female stutterers that differ from the negative stereotypes they hold for male stutterers. Although their stereotypes of both male and female stutterers incorporated the belief that stutterers are nervous and clumsy, their stereotypes of females contained allusions to insanity and gender confusion. That is, they described girls who were stutterers as insane and women who were stutterers as masculine. Their stereotypes of males contained no comparable allusions. The biased data base that describes the problem of stuttering as though it were a male problem probably accounts for such prejudices against female stutterers. When clinicians are trained by reading about the problems of *male* stutterers, hearing lectures about stuttering that represent it as a white, male problem, and providing clinical services almost exclusively to males, they are apt to conclude (consciously or unconsciously) that female stutterers are, to say the least, peculiar. They may consider them masculine because they exhibit a male problem and insane because they are masculine. At any rate, our biased data base, which presumably has contributed to such stereotypes of females, probably has led to unfortunate treatment experiences for females as such attitudes were projected to them. This may account for the fact that fewer women seek speech therapy than the gender ratio would suggest. Among adults, approximately 10 men seek treatment for each woman who does (Silverman & Zimmer, 1979). This ratio not only exceeds the typical ratio of approximately four men to one woman, but runs counter to the gender ratio describing adults' participation in health care services. Perhaps the gender ratio of stuttering in adulthood more closely resembles 10:1 than it does 4:1 since females tend to recover earlier than males (Seider, Gladstein & Kidd, 1983). But many girls who were treated by speech–language pathologists as though they were insane probably will not seek further contact with speech–language pathologists when they are adults.

This chapter summarizes research findings that describe the stuttering problems and speech therapy experiences female stutterers have had. The goal is to gently remind the reader that all clients, male and female, need to be approached as individuals and that individual problems need to be considered within the context of personal goals and ambitions and family and societal structures.

FEMALE STUTTERERS

Demographics

Prevalence

The ratio of male to female stutterers has been found to range from approximately 1.4:1 (Glasner & Rosenthal, 1957) to 10:1 (Schuell, 1946). Thus, it appears that more males than females are stutterers. But two recent observations challenge that conclusion. The first relates to a reported lag between the time a stuttering problem is diagnosed and the time treatment is begun, and the second is that elementary school classroom teachers are more likely to refer a boy for speech therapy who appears to have a stuttering problem than they are to refer a girl presenting an identical problem.

When asked to recall when they had first begun to stutter and when they subsequently began treatment, 10 adult female stutterers and 10 adult male stutterers reported different sequences. The women reported that they had begun to stutter noticeably, on the average, at 4.0 years of age and had entered treatment at 11.4 years. The men, however, reported that they had begun to stutter noticeably at 6.2 years and started therepy at 9.8 years (Silverman & Zimmer, 1982). Thus, the lag between the time the problem was perceived and the time treatment was initiated was more than twice as long for the women than it was for the men.

In 1980, Silverman and Van Opens (1980) surveyed suburban elementary classroom teachers to determine whether they showed a gender bias in their speech and language referals. The following anecdote was presented to 133 kindergarten through sixth-grade teachers, who were then asked to indicate how likely they would be to refer the child presenting the problem for speech-language therapy:

> Jimmy appears to be doing average written work but is often overlooked by his peers and is withdrawn conversationally. When he does speak, his speech is characterized by hesitation, 'uh's,' 'um's,' and syllable repetitions. This is especially promiment when he reads aloud.

Approximately half the teachers received this anecdote. The rest received an identical description of "Jenny's" problem. Eighty-sex percent reported that they would refer Jimmy, while 79% stated that they would refer Jenny. The difference was statistically significant at the 0.05 level of confidence.

These two observations challenge the reported sex ratio data. The sex ratio, remember, was derived from analyses of therapists' caseloads and from clinical records. Since it appears that both parents and classroom teachers believe that stuttering is a more serious problem for a boy than for a girl, and since they appear more willing to arrange for therapy for a boy than for a girl, the reported gender ratios based on clinical records may seriously underestimate the actual number of female stutterers of school age. Furthermore, since women with stuttering problems may be reluctant to seek therapy, the gender ratios based on analyses of clinical records of adults in treatment also may be biased, underestimating the number of adult females with stuttering problems. The sex-ratio may even equalize when all those with stuttering problems have the same chance of being referred for treatment and when prevalence data is based on surveys of populations by speech-language pathologists rather than on the records of speech-language pathologists.

The 1969 figure of 470,000 female stutterers living in the United States (based on data published by the National Advisory Neurological Diseases and Stroke Council, 1969) may have been only a rough estimate of the actual number of females with stuttering problems. (This figure would have to be up-dated to conform with current population data.)

Symptomatology

Symptomatology refers to those characteristics or features that comprise a disorder. The symptomatology of stuttering includes audible features, visible features, and attitudes.

Audible Features. Audible features are those behaviors identified as interjections of sounds; repetition of sounds, words, or phrases; revision of grammar or pronunciation; incomplete phrases; prolongations of sounds; unusually long, silent pauses; strangely patterned words or phrases where the rules of syllabification or timing seem to be disregarded; and sounds indicating extreme tension. These audible features have been collectively referred to as *stutterings* and, in some instances, as *disfluencies*.

Stutterings are found in the speech and oral reading of all peoples— children and adults (e.g., Williams, Silverman, & Kools, 1968); males and females (e.g., Johnson, 1961); stutterers and nonstutterers (e.g., Johnson, 1959, 1961); and English-speaking and non-English speaking peoples (e.g., Sasanuma, 1970). Some have tried to distinguish the stutterings of stutterers from the stutterings of nonstutterers. Believing that the stutterings of the two groups differ, the term *stutterings* has been used to describe stutterers' stutterings and the term disfluencies has been used to describe nonstutterers' stutterings. But Bloodstein (1981) has marshalled evidence showing that stutterings and disfluencies are members of the same response class—that is, both represent break-downs in serially ordered muscular behavior. Consequently, the term *stuttering* is used throughout this chapter to refer both to the stutterings of stutterers and the stutterings of nonstutterers. This is not to say that stutterers' stutterings are always the same as nonstutterers' stutterings. Stutterers' stutterings may be more forced on occasion, but not always. There are some stutterers who are labeled *interiorized* (Douglass & Quarrington, 1952), and these stutterers rarely stutter with noticeable tension. In fact, they rarely stutter. Their symptomatology consists primarily of the avoidance behaviors they have developed to keep themselves from stuttering. Extensive comparisons of stutterers' stutterings with non-stutterers' stutterings have shown that there is considerable overlap between the groups in terms of frequency of stuttering, distribution of stutterings within the speech sequence, and duration or extent of stutterings (Johnson, 1959, 1961; Williams, Silverman, & Kools, 1968, 1969a, 1969b). That is to say that most nonstutterers stutter about as much as most stutterers, and both groups' stutterings last about the same amount of time. Furthermore, both groups tend to stutter more at the beginnings of statements, on certain parts of speech—nouns, verbs, adjectives, and adverbs if adults, and pronouns, prepositions, conjunctions, and articles if children (Silverman, 1974; Helmreich & Bloodstein, 1973)—and on words of one syllable (Silverman, 1972b, 1978). Ironic as it seems, it appears that it is not the stutterings that distinguish stutterers from nonstutterers but, rather, fluent speech. The fluent speech of stutterers is thought to be slower and to contain more brief pauses than the fluent speech of nonstutterers (Prosek, Montgomery, Walden, & Schwartz, 1979; Zimmerman, 1980). This may be because stutterers have speech mechanisms that operate differently than those of non-stutterers, or because stutterers have learned to speak in a careful, precise manner to inhibit stuttering, or both. At any rate, it seems that stutterers' and nonstutterers' stutterings are more similar than different but that their fluent speech tends to differ.

Visible Features.   Visible features invariably stem from tense posturings of the facial musculature and/or musculature of the neck, thorax, abdomen, and, in some instances, the extremities as well. Persons with a stuttering problem may, when stuttering, forcibly compress their lips and flare their nostrils. They may swing their arm, stamp their foot, blink their eyes or squeeze them shut, turn their head from side to side, or tuck their chin into their chest. Some may adopt an expressionless, masklike countenance prior to and during speaking in order to avoid stuttering. There are many varieties of visible features possible, and all, including signs of agitation, stem from excess muscular tension. Some stutterers, as well as some nonstutterers, can be observed pacing to and fro before speaking to a group. At parties and in small groups, they may fold and unfold their arms across their chest, clasp and unclasp their hands, rock from side to side, or jiggle a foot or a leg.

Attitudes. There are certain attitudes or beliefs stutterers seem to have which, it can be argued, bring about the problem of stuttering in the first place and then serve to maintain it (Johnson, 1959; Sheehan, 1970). Among those attitudes are "Stuttering is bad," "It is wrong to stutter," "Only stutterers stutter," and "Stutterers differ from others because only stutterers stutter." It seems that when individuals accept the belief that it is wrong to do something, they will either (1) inhibit the behavior, or (2) exaggerate it, depending on the kind of recognition they are seeking. If they want approval and praise, they are apt to try to inhibit the behavior they consider bad. If they want to provoke negative attention and be punished, they probably will exaggerate the behavior. Once a decision has been reached, it generates behavior that reinforces it. For example, John, 4, notices that his parents grimace and turn away from him whenever he repeats a sound. If he cares deeply about winning their approval and praise, he probably will try to stop repeating sounds, or at least conceal the repeating he does. If, he notices that they object to his stuttering and if he has learned that the only way to get attention from them is to do something *wrong*, then he may stutter all the more openly.

Later in life many stutterers adopt a secondary set of beliefs revolving around the notion that only stutterers stutter. This tends to help them think of themselves as inferior to others, which may, in turn, spur them to adopt additional avoidance mannerisms, further embellishing the problem.

Attitudes are at the core of the problem: What a person thinks determines what he or she experiences.

Symptomatology of the Problem of Stuttering in Females. The symptomatology of female stutterers has received scant attention. Johnson published two major works, a study of the onset of stuttering (Johnson, 1959) and a study of the oral reading and speaking rates and stuttering behaviors of adult male and female stutterers (Johnson, 1961), and Sheehan coauthored a paper describing male and female stutterers' levels of aspiration (Sheehan & Zelen, 1955). The majority of the research appeared after 1970 (Kools & Berryman, 1971; Sheehan, 1979; Silverman, 1978, 1980, 1982; Silverman & Zimmer, 1975, 1976, 1979, 1982; Silverman, Zimmer, & Silverman, 1974). The findings of these studies can be summarized as follows:

1. Male and female stutterers show similar patterns of stuttering (Johnson, 1959, 1961; Kools & Berryman, 1971; Silverman & Zimmer, 1979), except that women produce fewer instances of revision and incomplete phrase, a difference that has been found to be statistically significant (Johnson, 1961; Silverman & Zimmer, 1979).

Females experiencing monthly menstrual cycles produce a significant increase in stuttering at premenstruation, when their frequency of stuttering at premenstruation is compared with their frequency of stuttering at ovulation (Silverman & Zimmer, 1976; Silverman, Zimmer, & Silverman, 1974). Premenstruation is the two or three days prior to the onset of menses when estrogen and progesterone levels drop markedly and feelings of tension and anxiety predominate (Ivey & Bardwick, 1968), while ovulation, approximately midcycle, is a time when there is a peak feeling of wellness.

2. Both men and women with stuttering problems appear basically well adjusted. On the *California Test of Personality* (Thrope, Clark & Tiegs, 1953), both groups scored around the fiftieth percentile overall (Silverman & Zimmer, 1979). The women, however, did score significantly higher than the men on the subtest of personal worth.

Men, however, show higher levels of aspiration than women, when level of aspiration is measured by comparing actual performance on the Rotter Board (a modified pin-ball device) with predicted performance (Sheehan & Zelen, 1955; Sheehan, 1979). In 1979, women's scores were higher than they were in 1955 (Sheehan, 1979).

3. Female stutterers appear less likely than male stutterers to avoid communicating. In their responses to the shortened form of Erickson's S-Scale (Andrews & Cutler, 1974; Erickson, 1969), the women appeared more confident than the men of their speaking ability and seemed to derive more pleasure from communicating (Silverman, 1982). The female stutterers did not, however, score as high as the nonstuttering female controls.

Treatment Experiences

Little research has been conducted to evaluate the responsiveness of female stutterers to treatment. The primary research is based on extensive interviewing of 10 adult female and 10 adult male stutterers (Silverman & Zimmer, 1982). It was discussed briefly in the introduction to this chapter and provides some tentative conclusions, given below. These are supported by more recent research (Sieder, Gladstien & Kidd, 1983) that has described the nature of recovery.

Onset of Treatment

Both the men and the women reported a lag from the time they were aware of having a problem to the time they recalled beginning treatment. But the lag for the women was almost twice as long as it was for the men. The women reported entering treatment, on the average, at 11.4 years—7.4 years after first being aware of having a stuttering problem. The men, in contrast, recalled entering treatment at 9.8 years—3.6 years after first becoming aware of having a stuttering problem. Although there was a sizable delay for both groups, there was a markedly longer delay for the women.

Treatment Effectiveness

Once they began treatment, the females, on the average, continued for a total of 2.8 nonconsecutive years. The men, in contrast, remained in treatment, on the average, for a total of 5.6 nonconsecutive years. These data suggest either that (1) the women's problems were remediated more swiftly than the men's because they were less serious than the men's or because the women were more highly motivated to change or (2) the women were less satisfied and quit prematurely.

Both the men and the women were unanimous in reporting that therapy was not helpful until they had graduated from high school. They said that once they had graduated and the choice of whether or not to attend speech therapy was theirs, they felt more cooperative and participated more fully. They were motivated to succeed because the decision to enter treatment had been their own.

There were some slight tendencies for the women to respond more positively to treatment modes that the men reported ineffective and vice versa. For example, some women preferred counseling and educational experiences, such as bibliotherapy, while several of the men prefered learning speech controls, although there was no clear demarcation between the groups. These tendencies were true for manner of treatment as well. While the women as a group expressed no particular preference for individual treatment as contrasted with group treatment, the men as a group showed a slight tendency to favor group treatment.

Recovery

While there have been several studies of recovery (e.g., Cooper, 1972; Shearer & Williams, 1965; Sheehan & Martyn, 1966; Wingate, 1964), only the recent report by Seider and her associates at the Yale University School of Medicine (Seider, Gladstien & Kidd, 1983) takes gender into account. Seider et al. reported that female stutterers tend to recover earlier and to be younger at onset of the problem.

Etiology

There does not seem to be any reason to believe that the cause of stuttering problems is any different for females than it is for males. As children, both females and males stutter about the same amount (Johnson, 1959) and in similar ways (e.g., Yairi, 1981). Boys, however, are exposed to greater pressure to produce fluent speech than are girls (Brownmiller, 1984; Schuell, 1946; Silverman & Van Opens, 1980). What this seems to mean is that environmental pressure in the form of sex-role stereotyping may play a significant role in the development of stuttering. (Johnson, 1959). Those caregivers who believe that stuttering is bad because it represents effeminacy in males or aggressiveness in females and who signal their children to stop stuttering are parents who are apt to have children who develop stuttering problems (Gray, 1940). No child develops a stuttering problem until he or she comes to believe that stuttering is bad. This point is well supported by a master's thesis completed at the University of Iowa under the direction of Wendell Johnson (Tudor, 1939). Johnson reportedly considered the data the strongest evidence he had in favor of the semantogenic, or diagnosogenic, theory of the onset of stuttering, but for reasons that shortly will be clear to the reader he suppressed the data during his lifetime.

Tudor selected six children, ages 5–15, who were living in an orphanage in Iowa, to serve as subjects. All were perfectly normal speakers. At the start of the experiment, she gave the following instructions to each child:

> The staff has come to the conclusion that you have a great deal of trouble with your speech. The types of interruptions which you have are very undesirable. These interruptions indicate stuttering. You have many of the symptoms of a child who is beginning to stutter. You must try to stop yourself immediately. Use your will power. Make up your mind that you are going to speak without a single interruption. It's absolutely necessary that you do this. Do anything to keep from stuttering. Try harder to speak fluently and evenly. If you have any interruptions, stop and begin again. Take a deep breath whenever you feel you are going to stutter. Don't ever speak unless you can do it right. You see how (the name of the child in the institution who stuttered rather severely) stutters, don't you? Well, he undoubtedly started the same way that you are starting. Watch your speech every minute and try to do something to improve it. Whatever you do speak fluently and avoid interruptions whatsoever in your speech (Tudor, 1939, pp. 10–11).

She then gave the following instructions to the teachers and matrons who interacted with the subjects:

> The staff has come to the conclusion that these children show definite symptoms of stuttering. The types of interruptions that they are having very frequently turn into stuttering. We have handled a number of cases very similar to these children. You should impress upon them the value of good speech, and that in order to have good speech one has to speak fluently. Watch their speech all the time very carefully and stop them when they have interruptions; stop them and have them say it over. Don't allow them to speak unless they can say it right. They should be made very conscious of their speech, and also they should be given opportunities to talk so that their mistakes can be pointed out to them.
>
> It is very important to watch for any changes in the child's personality, in his attitude toward his school work, in his attitude toward his playmates, etc. (Tudor, 1939, pp. 12–13).

She visited the orphanage once a month for 3 consecutive months to reinforce these ideas. At the end of four months, she described the children's speech as follows:

> All of the subjects . . . showed similar types of speech behavior during the experimental period. [First there was] a decrease in verbal output of all six subjects; that is, they were reluctant to speak and spoke only when they were urged to. Second, their rate of speaking was decreased. They spoke more slowly and with greater exactness. They had a tendency to weigh each word before they said it. Third, the length of response was shorter. The two younger subjects responded with one word whenever possible. Fourth, they all became more self-conscious. They appeared shy and embarrassed in many situations. Fifth, they accepted the fact that there was something definitely wrong with their speech. Sixth, every subject reacted to his speech interruptions in some manner. Some hung their heads; others gasped and covered their mouths with their hands; others laughed with embarrassment. In every case the children's behavior changed noticeably (Tudor, 1939, pp. 147–148).

Treatment was offered the children when the experiment concluded, but some effects lasted for years.

The preceding study is potent evidence that well-intentioned but misdirected adults may bring about stuttering problems in children who are developing normal speech. In the space of 3 months, children well past the age when the problem of stuttering typically begins became stutterers. They stuttered with exaggeration, they avoided speaking, and their self-concepts deteriorated. *All this happened despite the fact that teachers and matrons interacted with the children in ways they had been told would prevent the problem!* They monitored the children's speech for evidence of stuttering, thereby giving the children more attention than they had previously received and more attention than was given the other children. The more the children stuttered, the more attention they received. (For children who receive little personal attention, even criticism is better than benign neglect.) Moreoever, the children were instructed not to stutter. They were led to believe that their acceptance by the teachers and matrons depended upon whether or not they stopped stuttering. So, they struggled not to stutter, receiving even more attention for the struggle behavior. They quickly began to stutter with exaggeration, to avoid speaking, and to feel inadequate—all because well-intentioned adults believed that stuttering was a symptom of an emerging stuttering *problem* and that instructing the children not to stutter would prevent the problem from developing.

I believe that this is the basic mechanism responsible for the emergence of stuttering problems in both females and males, and I have elaborated elsewhere on what I believe to be the nature of the process (Silverman, 1984). The only difference that seems to be related to gender may be the "meaning" people ascribe to stuttering. Cultures and societies generally demand greater fluency from males than from females (e.g., Brownmiller, 1984; Schuell, 1946); therefore, families and teachers may make less of an effort to stop females from stuttering and more of an effort to stop males from stuttering (Silverman & Van Opens, 1980; Silverman & Zimmer, 1982).

ASSESSMENT STRATEGIES

Testing of female stutterers proceeds much along the same lines as the testing of male stutterers. For both, it is important to establish the kind of mental set that allows the client fully and freely to disclose personal information, which will bring about the greatest understanding of the individual and the problem. This means allowing clients freely to tell their stories as fully as necessary so that their "flavor" and "essence" can be absorbed. It is the flavor and essence of clients' stories that we want to capture during assessment so that we can individualize their treatment experiences. This means developing open protocols that are focused but nondirective, in contrast to closed protocols where clients are routinely administered the same battery of questions and subjected to the same methods of measurement. An open protocol may include a standard segment of questions and testing procedures to capture information helpful for research purposes, but clinical assessment requires that assessment procedures go beyond the routine. Each client needs to become known to the clinician as an individual with a particular set of concerns. Consequently, the suggestions that follow do not lend themselves to a rigid outline for assessment. Rather, they highlight areas and concerns that need to be probed to flesh out each client's story. Probably the major way that this particular section differs from similar sections in this book and in other books on stuttering and assessment is that this section includes suggestions for identifying gender-role stereotypes that may be contributing to the way a person stutters. These stereotypes may color the meaning of stuttering for the individual and contribute to particular avoidance patterns. Another way this section is different is that it makes suggestions to examine clients' language and communication patterns that correspond with gender-role stereotypes. These patterns may need to be targeted for change, depending on the client's personal goals.

Since age represents a critical variable in the assessment and management of the disorder, the suggestions offered are grouped into four subsections. Suggestions are given separately for preschoolers, elementary school children, adolescents, and adults. What follows reflects educated speculation about what ought to be done and how to go about it. This is based on awareness of research findings in the area of the psychology of gender differences in general and gender differences in communication, as well as personal observations from clinical experience. Although there are more suggestions for some ages than for others, this simply means that certain age groups are easier to assess from this standpoint than are others or that what was mentioned in a previous section also applies to those that follow.

Preschoolers

If parents have established a general pattern of concern about the adequacy of their child or the adequacy of their parenting or both, then when the child begins to stutter noticeably, they may become alarmed. This is especially likely to happen if they know someone with a stuttering problem. They may believe that the child's stuttering signifies the emergence of a stuttering problem, and, when they consult with a speech–language pathologist, they may approach the experience with a mixture of anxiety, fear, self-doubt, or guilt. These feelings will need to be addressed and dealt with in some fashion during the course of assessment, as will the child's feelings. The child will be aware of his or her parents' feelings at some level (Fraiberg, 1959) and may need to understand them, especially what they might mean about him or her.

The parents' gender-role expectations for themselves and for their child will have some bearing on the situation. These will need identification, analysis, and, in some instances, modification. For example, parents who believe males should be strong, which they may believe means being assertive and suppressing feelings, may be especially critial of their son's stuttering behavior, believing that stuttering is a sign of weakness and oversensitivity. If that is what they believe, they should be helped to understand that stuttering simply indicates that their son is being stressed and that criticizing him for stuttering is more likely to turn him into a stutterer than into a strong man. Likewise, parents who believe that females should be passive and submissive to authorities may believe that their daughter's stuttering signifies a form of aggression, an effort to control. They may criticize their daughter's stuttering to inhibit what they consider unfeminine behavior. They, too, will need to change their thinking about the meaning of stuttering, as criticism of their daughter's stuttering is more likely to cause a stuttering problem than to restore her femininity.

Assessment procedures involve three separate, yet related, activities: (1) *interviewing*, through which the clinician obtains information from the parents as well as the child that illuminates the present situation—information about the onset of the concern and how things have changed since then, the child's general health, the integrity of the family, the child's social experiences, and the family discipline practices; (2) *testing*, through which a direct assessment is made of the child's behavior, feelings, and attitudes; and (3) *counseling*, through which findings and recommendations are made to the family members, who are guided to carry out relevant problem solving. The following paragraphs expand on these ideas, giving some suggestions for ways to identify issues specific to gender.

Interviewing

An essential goal is to lead the parents into a description of family activities. Another is to discover expectations the parents have for their children. This information generally reveals gender-role stereotyping. Such stereotyping is harder to draw out in some families than in others. For example, it is especially difficult to obtain narrative accounts of child-rearing practices from parents who are either in awe of the superior position or education of the clinician or resentful of the clinician's position of authority. Parents who feel guilty because they believe they have caused their child's problems may be reluctant to talk about their child-rearing practices. With these parents, the best the clinician can hope to do is to communicate a willingness to listen uncritically to their story. This can be communicated by speech, saying such things as, "Help me understand how you respond to Denise's stuttering so that I can have a better feeling for your concerns," "How can I help you today?'' ''Tell me what I can do for you,'' and ''Tell me what's troubling you.'' A nonjudgmental attitude also can be communicated by tone of voice, facial expression, posture, gestures, rate of speech, and even apparel (Bernstein, Bernstein, & Dana, 1970; Evans, Hearn, Uhlemann, & Ivey, 1979). In fact, as much as 93% of what we communicate is nonverbal (Mehrabian, 1971).

Sucessful interviewing—creating free communication flow between clinician and client—depends on several ingredients:

1. *Developing appropriate structure*. It is important to develop a pocket in space and time where people feel safe, supported, and directed. This means that the clinician needs to attend not only to the physical characteristics of the room or rooms in which the encounter takes place, such as lighting, ventilation, color, appointments, positioning of the furniture, and type of furniture (Myers & Myers, 1980), but also to communiating clearly at the outset the purpose and plan of the encounter.

2. *Conveying interest, warmth, and a caring attitude*. Unless clients feel the clinician cares about them as people, they are apt to withhold information about beliefs and behaviors that might be criticized. The best way to convey genuine regard for clients is to feel it, to approach the interview with the intent to help them help themselves by clarifying the situation in which they presently find themselves and identifying possible options.

3. *Being professional*. This relates to the other two ingredients. It means conveying a sense of competency by being prompt, well groomed, extroverted, and positive. It also implies being comfortable with oneself and accepting of others.

Testing

Testing can be approached either directly or indirectly. Observation is another name for indirect testing, where the child is observed interacting with parents or other caregivers and, if possible, with playmates. This is done, preferably, in everyday situations, to identify the way the parties interact. This reveals what the child is experiencing and how he or she functions under the circumstances. It also conveys attitudes toward gender roles. For example, Evelyn and Marvin might be observed coaching 4-year-old Gavin to be verbally aggressive around boys because they believe that to be quiet is a sign of weakness in a male. Being verbally aggressive may be contrary to Gavin's gentle nature. Maura's parents, on the other hand, may insist that Maura behave in a passive, demure manner around others, yet Maura may be strong willed and assertive. Both Gavin and Maura may stutter with greater frequency and exaggeration around their parents because of the conflict they experience between wanting to express themselves honestly and wanting to behave in ways that please their parents (Sheehan, 1970).

Observing parent–child interactions also provides direct information about whether or not parents encourage their child's explorations, that is, whether they encourage the child's development of autonomy or seek instead the child's conformance to their beliefs. These observations similarly reveal the discipline practices of the parents and the child's reactions to them. Finally, they exemplify the way the parents speak to their child; that is, do they speak softly and slowly using a vocabulary their child can understand or do they talk *at* their child and over his or her head (Saltz, Campbell, & Skotko, 1983)?

More direct testing to establish the integrity of the speech and hearing mechanism and to identify linguistic and cognitive skill development and verbal fluency can also reveal added information about the child's perception of expected sex role behaviors. For example, 3-year-old Sara is instructed to draw a picture of how she feels while she is stuttering. When questioned about the drawing, Sara reports that she feels bad because "girls aren't supposed to talk that way." This provides one more piece of evidence that Sara and her caregivers consider stuttering bad because they see it as unfeminine. Similar kinds of information may be revealed during the administration of an articulation test or a test of syntactic functioning.

Counseling

The belief that stuttering is detrimental to one's masculinity or femininity needs to be addressed. Caregivers need to be helped to see that stuttering behavior—interjections, part-word repetitions, whole-word repetitions, phrase repetitions, revisions, incomplete phrases, broken words, prolongations, tense pauses, and unfilled pauses—is commonplace among preschoolers (Silverman, 1973b; Yairi, 1981). Most preschoolers stutter at the beginnings of utterances; on pronouns, such as *I, we,* and *you,* conjunctions, prepositions, and articles—words they often use to initiate their utterances; and on words of one syllable (Silverman, 1972a; 1972b; 1974). They also tend to stutter when they feel pressured to communicate (Silverman, 1973b). When they do stutter, their stutterings tend to occur in clusters, or volleys, of two or more (Silverman, 1973a).

Stuttering indicates that the child is being stressed, that is, feeling pressured to perform quickly and accurately enough to satisfy caregivers. The caregivers' role, then, is to identify stressors and to remove or defuse them (Zwitman, 1978). This includes, when necessary, a change in attitude regarding what stuttering implies about the child's gender identity and intelligence.

Elementary School Children

Interviewing involves the child directly and uncovers the child's feelings and beliefs about speaking and communicating. With younger children, this can be accomplished through the use of puppets, human figures in home, school, and play settings, drawings, and pictures. Older children can be asked to express their feelings and beliefs. Care needs to be taken, however, that the clinician does not plant suggestions to the child that become self-fulfilling prophecies (Williams, 1970).

Testing measures the effectiveness of the speech and hearing mechanism and all oral communication skills. Oral reading should be sampled as should narrative speech. The clinician needs to ascertain if the child is avoiding communication in order to conceal stuttering, and if so, in what ways. Avoidances may take the form of talking less, avoiding certain people and situations, and using word substitutions as well as starters and postponers.

The clinician will also want to note the extent to which torso rigidity and breathing irregularities occur. These generally indicate that the child is suffering from fear and anxiety (Versteegh-Vermeij, 1984). Poor eye contact, concaved (slumped) posture, and other signs of diminishing self-esteem and withdrawal need to be acknowledged. Assessment of language usage and conversational style can help identify the extent to which the child is establishing a stereotypic gender-role (Lynch, 1983). For example, suppose you experienced the following dialogue with a nine-year-old boy:

> Clinician: Tell me, Aaron, do you like talking with your classmates?
> Aaron: Nope.
> Clinician: What's the problem?
> Aaron: I—well, they um, laugh at me.
> Clinician: Laugh at you!
> Aaron: Yeah, th, the, the (cheeks puffing up, eyes widening), they think I'm stupid.
> Clinician: Stupid!
> Aaron: Yeah, th, th, th, they th-th-th-think buh, buh, buh, boys shouldn't stutter.

Apparently, Aaron's classmates ridicule Aaron for being less of a boy because he stutters with exaggeration. It seems from this short exchange that Aaron may be beginning to accept their belief that boys should not stutter.

A dialogue with Marcia, in contrast, revealed she felt rejected because her stuttering was considered inappropriate behavior for a girl:

> Marcia: I really don't want to talk about it.
> Clinician: It hurts a lot, huh?
> Marcia: Yeah, (Long pause.) It really isn't fair that they laugh at me just because I stutter.
> Clinician: Stuttering isn't funny.
> Marcia: I know, but they think girls shouldn't talk that way. It's unfeminine—you know, with my tongue sticking out and all.
> Clinician: What do you think about that?
> Marcia: Well, I ehhhh (long pause while staring fixedly at the clinician—articulators are locked into position for "eh," and the torso is rigid, impeding deep and flowing respiration) ehh duh, don't think it makes a difference, but my sisters say girls don't do those things. My parents think it's wrong too. I can tell from the way they look at me—like I'm a freak or something.

Marcia, 10, is beginning to question her femininity and ultimately her self-worth because she stutters with exaggeration.

When counseling the child and the parents, the clinician needs to share information relative to the nature of stuttering, that is, that stutterings are speech mistakes everyone makes from time to time; that they are neither good nor bad—they simply are; that it is possible to stutter *easily*, without excess tension and forcing—the way others do; and that it doesn't mean that you are less of a girl or less of a boy if you stutter. Teachers and others who come into regular contact with the child may also need to hear this from the clinician.

Adolescents

Most adolescents with a stuttering problem have been experiencing failure in speech therapy for some time and, consequently, may be unenthusiastic about continuing treatment (Silverman & Zimmer, 1982). They may come to therapy out of a sense of obligation to their parents, teachers, or themselves to "do something" about their speech, but they may, at the same time, think they are hopeless or that therapy is worthless or both.

Assessment needs to establish the adolescent's motives for entering treatment, his or her expectations regarding the outcome of treatment, and his or her degree of openness to work on attitudes as well as speech behaviors. Unless attitudes toward stuttering and oneself as a speaker become realistic and harmonious, it is unlikely that lasting change will be experienced (Andrews, Guitar, & Howie, 1980; Sugarmen, 1979).

Males and females may have different preferences for therapy activities (instrumental aids, speech controls, and/or altering attitudes); for the general delivery of services (whether therapy is conducted in an individual, group, or mixed format and whether the groups are homogeneous or heterogeneous); and for the gender of the clinician (Silverman & Zimmer, 1982).

Beyond that, adolescents require no different consideration than elementary school children and preschoolers. If the outcome of assessment is to recommend treatment and the adolescent is willing to enter into a treatment relationship, then a contract should be negotiated among the adolescent, the therapist, and those legally responsible for the adolescent (Myers, 1983).

Adults

Adults frequently are propelled to seek change—when they feel stuck in a job or a particular lifestyle and want to break free—but, occasionally, they enter therapy to seek refuge or to play out games that sabotage change. Consider the following example from Hornyak's 1980 article in *Asha* entitled, "The Rescue Game and The Speech–Language Pathologist" (Hornyak, 1980):

> A person contacts a speech–language pathologist and requests help for his stuttering problem. The speech–language pathologist accepts the client and the therapy process starts. The early sessions seem to progress smoothly and the client and speech–language pathologist develop a 'friendly' relationship. The client's nonfluency may lessen considerably during these sessions. However, outside the clinic, the client's behavior does not change. The speech–language pathologist eventually becomes aware of this and puts pressure on the client to do outside assignments and to try harder. As more pressure is put on the client, she/he begins to cancel sessions due to illness, work, or other 'good' reasons. Finally she/he stops coming. (p. 86)

To avoid such unpleasant and nonproductive experiences for both the client and the clinician, it is important to identify underlying motives related to seeking therapy. Obtaining a thorough record of the individual's previous treatment experiences along with an account of what was successful and what was not and why can be very helpful.

It is possible that more males than females may seek treatment (Silverman & Zimmer, 1979). Women who do seek treatment may, in general, prefer individual treatment as opposed to group treatment (Silverman & Zimmer, 1982). Research has shown that women in mixed—male and female—instructional and discussion groups tend to feel ignored and sometimes resented, leading them to restrict their participation to an occasional comment now-and-then (Thorne & Henley, 1975). Perhaps women with stuttering problems feel similarly when they enter mixed treatment groups.

TREATMENT

There is very little data describing the interaction between a client's gender and his or her responsiveness to treatment procedures. That which is available pertains to the experiences of adolescents and adults. The section below allotted to preschoolers and elementary school children represents reasoned speculation. The suggestions in that section stem from personal experience and awareness of child development.

Preschoolers and Elementary School Children

Girls may be less willing to experiment than boys (Maccoby & Jacklin, 1975). Consequently, girls in treatment may need more encouragment than boys to try different ways of stuttering. They may be willing to try easier methods of stuttering if they can first teach such methods to a doll or puppet. Taking the role of teacher, mother, or clinician, while stereotypic, may make the learning of easier ways of stuttering more appealing.

Girls also may be more responsive in individual than in group treatment. Adolescent girls are more responsive in individual therapy (Godenne, 1982), and it may be that such a preference manifests itself as early as the preschool years. A preference for individual treatment is consistent with some of Gilligan's research (e.g., Gilligan, 1982). Gilligan has reported that girls do not like to play games in which there are winners and losers. She reported that girls prefer connectedness and affiliation to competetiveness. Consequently, in treatment groups viewed as competitive, girls may withdraw to a point where they benefit little.

Adolescents and Adults

Adolescents enrolled in psychotherapy have been described as erratic in attendance and unwilling to make long-term commitments to treatment (Richmond & Gaines, 1979). Adults, when recollecting their therapy experiences as adolescents, report having had a lack of faith in and understanding of the treatment process (Silverman & Zimmer, 1982). They explained that they had difficulty understanding both their role and that of the therapist, stating that it was not until they were adults and willing to take responsibility for change that they were ready to take full advantage of therapy. This was true for both the males and the females.

Other than the Silverman & Zimmer (1982) data, there is little information about stutterers' impressions of the therapy process or stutterers' preferences for certain treatment features. Silverman & Zimmer (1982) reported that the 10 adult females they interviewed showed a slight preference for individual treatment. The 10 males showed no clear preference for one therapy mode over another. Neither the females nor the males expressed a preference for a therapist of the same or the opposite gender. Females were just as likely to state they preferred working with a female therapist as with a male therapist, and so were male stutterers.

Both the male and the female stutterers interviewed reported that they preferred working with a therapist who was patient, warm, empathetic, and personal and found it difficult to work with a therapist who possessed the traits they described as superiority, insensitivity, and pushiness and who seemed uninvolved and authoritarian.

There was a slight difference, however, in the needs of female stutterers as compared to males stutterers regarding the direction taken in treatment. Females seem to value highly attitude-normalization types of activities, while males seem to prefer learning speech controls. Since twice as many male stutterers (six) as female stutterers in the Silverman & Zimmer (1982) study received some type of personal counseling, males apparently value attitude normalization work but may prefer to undertake such activity with counselors rather than with speech–language therapists.

Communication skill development also may need to be approached differently with females. Lynch (1983), in a review paper in *Asha*, outlined the different ways males and females use language as well as the different ways people use language to refer to males and females. She concluded, "gender related differences in language share characteristics with the linguistic expression of dominance and/or power" (p. 42).

Applied to female stutterers, this suggests that giving up the role of stutterer (Sheehan, 1970) might require learning more assertive, potent, and authoritative conversational styles. The woman who gives up the role of stutterer, no longer wishing to be seen as passive and powerless, may demand assistance learning to communicate differently. This puts pressure on the therapist to become familiar with linguistic and stylistic variables associated with displays of power and dominance. Consider the situation of Mary Arnold (fictitious name), a 25-year-old, successfully learning to stutter fluently by reducing her overall speech rate and prolonging continuants. She fears that her new fluent speaking behavior may be jeopardized should she continue to interact passively.

Clinician: Tell me more about what you want.

Mary: I want to learn to speak in such a way that I appear confident, sure of myself, in charge and grounded. I don't want to be a wimp.

Clinician: But you are doing fine learning to stutter fluently . . .

Mary: Yes, but that's not enough. Now that my speech is good I want to learn to communiate well enough to get the breaks I know I'm ready for. I don't want to be overlooked. I want to be noticed as someone who counts, someone who has something important to say, someone worth listening to. Like you, for instance. . . . I want to sound as sure of myself as you do. I want to speak clearly like you do. I have all these old habits of not talking and of speaking as little as possible. I really need to learn to take turns in a conversation. I'd always be thinking about myself instead of paying attention to others, and I never really noticed others that much—too turned inward, I guess. I feel like a klutz around others. I don't feel good just pastiming, you know, just talking to people 'cause I never really learned how—always been too busy trying to avoid stuttering. Now I don't stutter the way I used to, and that's good, but now I want to be able to TALK the way others do, and I don't know how, and if I don't learn, I'll just end up standing around like a dumbell at parties, and I won't do any better at work!

The clinician must decide how to deal with Mary's requests. They mirror the needs of many stutterers, whether or not they are as articulate and as forthright as Mary. Once adolescents and adults learn to stutter fluently, they often recognize that they are deficient in interpersonal communication skills and that they need to learn those skills if they are to reach their goals as successful communicators. The clinician, responding to Mary's request needs to utilize her knowledge of the well-established gender differences in communication. Females may benefit from learning to use vocal pitch, intonation patterns, vocabulary, and syntax (Kraemer, 1974) to convey self-assurance and potency. When they participate in group discussions, they also need to learn to handle the inevitable interruptions and signs of disinterest that others may display (Thorne & Henley, 1975). For example, I attended a meeting of a regional self-help group for adult stutterers in which approximately 14 adults took part: about 10 males and four females. A male served as discussion leader. The males all spoke with the assurance that what they had to say was worthwhile, and their confidence seemed to grow as their contributions were affirmed by the others. When the females spoke, the attitude of the group changed abruptly. People became more quiet, but not in an attentive way. The quiet seemed to exemplify the thought that "we must be patient while she says what is on her mind, and then we can get back to the real business of the group." Their reactions were less affirming and more skeptical. After a short time, the group appeared impatient and gave nonverbal signals that the speaker should finish—something that was rarely done while a man was talking. When a woman completed her contribution, an attitude of relief seemed to be expressed by the group, communicating, "Well, now that's over and we can get back to the *real* business."

Clinicians need to welcome females sincerely into treatment groups, giving them the same privileges and responsibilities that they give males. Females should be given as fair an opportunity as males to be heard and to have their contributions valued. This may require the clinician's encouragement and respect. That is, the clinician should call on females as enthusiastically as males and provide them with the same sort of feedback. The therapist is a key force in group treatment and cannot simply sit back and wait for the group to welcome and incorporate female members on its own.

Negative stereotypic attitudes clinicians may have about female stutterers can be detrimental in other ways. On the one hand, females who detect that the clinician believes "women have their place" may either decline to enter a treatment relationship with that particular clinician or may overgeneralize and refuse to enter treatment with *any* speech-language pathologist. On the other hand, believing that any therapy is better than none, a female stutterer may enroll in a treatment program even though she believes the clinician has a gender-bias. Under those circumstances, it is unlikely that constructive change will occur. This would be due to several factors: a less than whole-hearted commitment to the program because of feelings of alienation from the therapist; spending more energy on resentment than on change because she believes the therapist is "holding out" on her; and receiving less direction and encouragement from the therapist who really does not believe women have a right to realize their full potential as human beings.

Sometimes speech–language therapy is not enough for a particular client. Some clients may benefit from the communication skills they can learn as a member of a Toastmaster's club or by taking a Dale Carnegie course. Others may benefit from support groups, such as those sponsored by the National Council of Adult Stutterers and the National Stuttering Project. Some may wish to take assertiveness training and workshops on empowerment. Some may be so troubled by personal concerns that they have little energy to put into changing their speech and may be candidates for psychotherapy or personal counseling.

The following transcript is excerpted from a therapy session a graduate student conducted with a young, adult male stutterer. It exemplifies the kinds of cues a stutterer sends when he or she is too troubled by personal concerns to fully participate in treatment:

Clinician: Did you—have you been trying to do those—the cancellation techniques at all?

Client: Uh, when I remember about it, yeah.

Clinician: Like in what situations have you—can you give me any examples?

Client: Well, un, well, um, I'm alone when I'm doing it, and like if I'm reading something, then I do it, and usually when I do think about it, you know, like I'm talking to people, uh, in class, when it comes to mind. It comes right after I say something.

Clinician: Okay.

Client: You know, 'cause I'm just not, uh used to it yet.

Clinician: Right, it takes some time. It definitely takes some-time. I agree. Okay, today as it does take some time, we're going to spend a lot of time on it. And I want you to pull out the paper that you wrote on explaining what to do when you cancel and some of the different ways of canceling.

Client: You mean this one here?

Clinician: Yes, you wrote those out. Okay. Tell me what a
            cancellation is. Tell me in your own words why you
            think you're doing this technique, what it is, and
            then tell me about the two ways you wrote down
            to do it.

Client: Let's see. Tell me in—tell you in my, uh, my, uh,
            my own words. What? What did you say?

Clinician: Tell me in your own words what a cancellation is,
            why do you think you are doing it, what good it
            does for you.

Client: Um, well, first off, uh, it's, uh, you're to speak
            more fluent, uh, and like, um. . . .

Clinician: How does it help you speak more fluently?

Client: Well, like if I'm go—or like when coming up on a
            word I'm pretty sure that I'm gonna stutter and,
            you know, I stop there and then I say the word in
            myself and I say the word aloud.

Clinician: That's one way of doing it. Right. That's how
            it. . . .

Client: You can say, uh, see I was gonna go over this stuff
            here, but, see, I found out last week Saturday my
            grandfather is in the midst of, uh, with cancer.
            They're trying to find a nursing home for him, you
            know, and like, uh, and like, uh, if they'll be com-
            ing up to the house tonight, then, uh, uh, yeah—
            so, that's been on my mind pretty much of the
            time, you know, so, uh, uh, I was gon—and I was
            gonna, gonna go. In fact, every time that I thought
            about it, you know, uh, ih, ih, it ended up being
            so late, you know, that I just wanted, wanted to
            go to bed, like, I started doing, doing it last night.
            It was about, about 11:30—quarter, uh, quarter, uh,
            tuh, wh—quarter to twelve. You know I was,
            was—I was, I mean, I'm going over it and, and,
            and, and, and, and, and, and and, my eyes started
            to shut. I thought, 'Go to bed; go to bed.'

Clinician: Yeah, you're right.

Client: I'll do it, though, in the morning.

Clinician: Well, you know, do try to get a chance to do it.
            Maybe this weekend would be good, when you're

	sitting around, maybe, uh, you know what would be better is when you wake up in the morning, probably.
Client:	'Cause, un, uh, it's, uh, see it ta—it takes, uh, like this morning, well, the, uh, desk called me at 5:30, you know, uh, for an alarm. My dad called me at about quarter to six, and I didn't get, get, get up until 6:30.
Clinician:	Oh, okay, well, maybe on like Saturday or Sunday morning you could get up maybe 15 minutes early 'cause you don't have to be a lot of different places on the weekend.
Client:	Yeah, I don't.
Clinician:	So, then, you know, you could get up and try to go over . . .
Client:	But, uh, when I went to Basic Skills today, uh, we got an asa, asa, as, assignment in there. What the heck that she, that she, that she giving us this stuff for? I don't know—I wouldn't know, but you know, and, and, and, then I sa, I sa, I was like, man, I was . . .
Clinician:	I want you to tell me about this, but I want you to cancel in your speech.

This exchange was not atypical for this client. He frequently reiterated some personal crisis to explain why he could not work on his speech. It was clear that he wanted to come to treatment because his attendance was excellent, but it was equally clear that he did not want to do anything to change. Further counseling was necessary to help him resolve this conflict.

THE CHALLENGE OF THE FEMALE STUTTERER

Recognizing the existence of the female stutterer forces us as a profession and as individuals to examine more closely our knowledge of stuttering problems and our attitudes toward working with people who present those problems. The few studies that have described the symptomatology and experiences of female stutterers have shown that we cannot as a profession continue to think that only by describing the symptoms and experiences of male stutterers can we know all we need to know about the problem of stuttering. For instance, the Silverman and Van Opens data (Silverman & Van Opens, 1980) showing that teachers consider the problem of stuttering more serious for a boy than for a girl challenges us to reconsider both the potency of environmental factors in the formation of stuttering problems and the general inaccuracy of referral systems. The Silverman and Zimmer (1982) data show that females respond differently to treatment options than males. All in all, it seems we need to reevaluate our data and assumptions.

As clinicians we need to open ourselves more fully to female stutterers. We need to disabuse ourselves of notions we may have that female stutterers are insane or masculine because they have a "male" problem. The problem of stuttering represents unsuccessful coping strategies, nothing more and nothing less. We can help both females and males learn to substitute new speaking behaviors for old. To do this, we need to consider carefully the needs, the strengths, and the weakness of all our clients and to abandon whatever stereotypes we may have about stutterers that only serve to limit them and us.

REFERENCES

Andrews, G., & Cutler, J. (1974). The relation between changes in symptom level and attitudes. *Journal of Speech and Hearing Disorders, 39*, 312–319.
Andrews, G., Guitar, B., & Howie, P. (1980). Meta-analysis of the effects of stuttering treatment. *Journal of Speech and Hearing Disorders, 45*, 287–307.
Bernstein, L., Bernstein, R., & Dana, R. (1970). *Interviewing: A guide for health professionals* (2nd ed.). New York: Appleton-Century-Crofts.
Bloodstein, O. (1981). *A handbook on stuttering*. Chicago: National Easter Seal Society.
Brownmiller, S. (1984). *Femininity*. New York: Linden.
Cooper, E. (1972). Recovery from stuttering in a junior and senior high school population. *Journal of Speech and Hearing Research, 15*, 632–638.
Douglass, E., & Quarrington, B. (1952). The differentiation of interiorized and exteriorized secondary stuttering. *Journal of Speech and Hearing Disorders, 17*, 377–385.
Erickson, R. (1969). Assessing communication attitudes among stutterers. *Journal of Speech and Hearing Research, 3*, 181–186.
Evans, D., Hearn, M., Uhlemann, M., & Ivey, A. (1979). *Essential interviewing*. Monterey, CA: Brooks/Cole.
Fraiberg, S. (1959). *The magic years*. New York: Charles Scribner's Sons.
Gilligan, C. (1982). *In a different voice*. Cambridge, MA: Harvard University Press.
Glasner, P., & Rosenthal, D. (1957). Parental diagnosis of stuttering in young children. *Journal of Speech and Hearing Disorders, 22*, 288–295.
Godenne, G. (1982). The adolescent girl and her female therapist. *Adolescence, 17*, 225–242.
Gray, M. (1940). The X family: A clinical and laboratory study of a "stuttering" family. *Journal of Speech Disorders, 5*, 343–348.

Helmreich, H., & Bloodstein, O. (1973). The grammatical factor in childhood disfluency in relation to the continuity hypothesis. *Journal of Speech and Hearing Research, 16,* 731–738.

Horynak, A. (1980). The rescue game and the speech–language pathologist. *Asha, 22,* 86–89.

Ivey, M., & Bardwick, J. (1968). Patterns of affective fluctuation during the menstrual cycle. *Psychosomatic Medicine, 30,* 336–345.

Johnson, W. (1959). *The onset of stuttering.* Minneapolis: The University of Minnesota Press.

Johnson, W. (1961). Measurement of oral reading and speaking rate and disfluency of adult male and female stutterers and nonstutterers. *Journal of Speech and Hearing Disorders, Monogr. Suppl. 7,* 1–20.

Kools, J. & Berryman, J. (1971). Differences in disfluency behavior between male and female nonstuttering children. *Journal of Speech and Hearing Research, 14,* 125–130.

Kraemer, C. (1974). Folk-linguistics: Wishy washy mommy talk. *Psychology Today, 6,* 82–85.

Lynch, J. (1983). Gender differences in language. *Asha, 25,* 37–42.

Maccoby, E., & Jacklin, E. (1974). *The psychology of sex differences.* Standford, CA: Standford University Press.

Mehrabian, A. (1971). *Silent messages.* Belmont, CA: Wadsworth.

Myers, J. (1983). Legal issues surrounding psychotherapy with minor clients. *Transactional Analysis Journal, 13,* 182–189.

Myers, G., & Myers, M. (1980). *The dynamics of human communication* (3rd ed.). New York: McGraw-Hill.

NINDS, (1969). *Human Communication and Its Disorders.—An Overview.* Bethesda, Maryland: U.S. Department of Health, Education, and Welfare.

Prosek, R., Montgomery, A., Walden, B., & Schwartz, D. (1979). Reaction-time measures of stutterers and nonstutterers. *Journal of Fluency Disorders, 4,* 215–222.

Richmond, L., & Gaines, T. (1979). Factors influencing attendance in group psychotherapy with adolescents. *Adolescence, 14,* 715–720.

Saltz, E., Campbell, S., & Skotko, D. (1983). Verbal control of behavior: The effects of shouting. *Developmental Psychology, 19,* 461–464.

Sasanuma, S. (1968). *A description of the disfluent speech behavior of stuttering and nonstuttering Japanese children.* Unpublished Ph.D. dissertation, The University of Iowa.

Schuell, H. (1946). Sex differences in relation to stuttering. Part I. *Journal of Speech Disorders, 11,* 277–298.

Seider, R., Gladstien, K., & Kidd, K. (1983). Recovery and persistence of stuttering among relatives of stutterers. *Journal of Speech and Hearing Disorders, 48,* 402–408.

Shearer, W., & Williams, J. (1965). Self-recovery from stuttering. *Journal of Speech and Hearing Disorders, 30,* 288–290.

Sheehan, J. (1970). *Stuttering: Research and therapy.* New York: Harper & Row.

Sheehan, J. (1979). Level of aspiration in female stutterers: Changing times? *Journal of Speech and Hearing Disorders, 44,* 479–486.

Sheehan, J., & Martyn, M. (1966). Spontaneous recovery from stuttering. *Journal of Speech and Hearing Research, 9,* 121–135.

Sheehan, J., & Zelen, S. (1955). Level of aspiration in stutterers and nonstutterers. *Journal of Abnormal Social Psychology, 51,* 83–86.

Silverman, E.-M. (1972a). Generality of disfluency data collected from preschoolers. *Journal of Speech and Hearing Research, 15,* 84–92.

Silverman, E.-M. (1972b). Preschoolers' speech disfluency: Single-syllable word repetition. *Perceptual Motor Skills, 35,* 1002.

Silverman, E.-M. (1973a). Clustering: A characteristic of preschoolers' speech disfluency. *Journal of Speech and Hearing Research, 16,* 578–583.

Silverman, E.-M. (1973b). The influence of preschoolers' speech usage on their disfluency frequency. *Journal of Speech and Hearing Research, 16,* 474–481.

Silverman, E.-M. (1974). Word position and grammatical function in relation to preschoolers' speech disfluency. *Perceptual Motor Skills, 39,* 267–272.

Silverman, E.-M. (1978). Adults' speech disfluency: Single-syllable word repetition. *Perceptual Motor Skills, 46,* 970.

Silverman, E.-M. (1980). Communication attitudes of women who stutter. *Journal of Speech and Hearing Disorders, 45,* 533–539.

Silverman, E.-M. (1982). Speech–language clinicians' and university students' impressions of women and girls who stutter. *Journal of Fluency Disorders, 7,* 469–478.

Silverman, E.-M. (1984). *Stuttering. Detection and prevention. Treatment for children, adolescents, and adults.* Unpublished manuscript.

Silverman, E.-M., & Van Opens, K. (1980). An investigation of sex-bias in classroom teachers' speech and language referrals. *Language, Speech, and Hearing Services in the Schools, 11,* 169–174.

Silverman, E.-M., & Zimmer, C. (1975). Speech fluency fluctuations during the menstrual cycle. *Journal of Speech and Hearing Research, 18,* 202–206.

Silverman, E.-M., & Zimmer, C. (1976). Replication of "Speech fluency fluctuations during the menstrual cycle." *Perceptual Motor Skills, 42,* 1004–1006.

Silverman, E.-M., & Zimmer, C. (1979). Women who stutter: Personality and speech characteristics. *Journal of Speech and Hearing Research, 22,* 553–564.

Silverman, E.-M., & Zimmer, C. (1982). Demographic characteristics and treatment experiences of women and men who stutter. *Journal of Fluency Disorders, 7,* 273–285.

Silverman, E.-M., Zimmer, C., & Silverman, F. (1974). Variability in stutterers' disfluency: The menstrual cycle. *Perceptual Motor Skills, 38,* 1037–1038.

Sugarman, M. (1979). From being a stutterer to becoming a person who stutters. *Transactional Analysis Journal, 9,* 41–44.

Thorne, B., & Henley, N. (Eds.) (1975). *Language and sex: Difference and dominance.* Rowley, MA: Newbury House.

Thorpe, L., Clark, W., & Tiegs, E. (1953). *California test of personality (manual).* Monterey, CA: California Test Bureau.

Tudor, M. (1939). *An experimental study of the effect of evaluative labeling on speech fluency.* Unpublished master's thesis, The University of Iowa, Iowa City, IA.

Versteegh-Vermeij, E., (1984). Body, concept, self concept and balance. In J. Gruss (Ed.), *Stuttering therapy: Transfer and maintenance* (pp. 75–86). Memphis, TN: Speech Foundation of America.

Williams, D. (1970). Stuttering therapy with children. In L. Travis (Ed.), *Handbook of speech pathology and audiology* (pp. 1073–1094). New York: Appleton-Century-Crofts.

Williams, D., Silverman, F., & Kools, J. (1968). Disfluency behavior of elementary-school stutterers and nonstutterers: The adaptation effect. *Journal of Speech and Hearing Research, 11,* 622–630.

Williams, D., Silverman, F., & Kools, J. (1969a). Disfluency behavior of elementary school stutterers and nonstutterers: The consistency effect. *Journal of Speech and Hearing Research, 12,* 301–307.

Williams, D., Silverman, F., & Kools, J. (1969b). Disfluency behavior of elementary school stutterers and nonstutterers: Loci of instances of disfluency. *Journal of Speech and Hearing Research, 12,* 308–318.

Wingate, M. (1964). Recovery from stuttering. *Journal of Speech and Hearing Disorders, 29,* 312–321.

Yairi, E. (1981). Disfluencies of normally speaking two-year-old children. *Journal of Speech and Hearing Research, 24,* 490–495.

Zimmerman, G. (1980). Stuttering: A disorder of movement. *Journal of Speech and Hearing Research, 23,* 122–136.

Zwitman, D. (1978). *The disfluent child.* Baltimore, MD: University Park Press.

4

The Exceptionally Severe Stutterer

Pat Richard Sacco

INTRODUCTION

This chapter discusses the problems associated with the exceptionally severe stutterer. This individual is readily identified as exceptionally severe by extremes in some or all of those criteria usually employed in the assessment process, namely, frequency and duration of stuttering, and physical concomitants of the above (Riley, 1980).

A great deal of research has been done in the area of stuttering during the last decade, representing more than one-fourth of the total of our knowledge in stuttering (Bloodstein, 1981). Yet, there are data (St. Louis & Lass, 1980, 1981) that students in speech–language pathology still regard stuttering as a mysterious and not well-understood disorder. Andrews, Craig, Feyer, Hoddinott, Howie & Neilson (1983) have countered that individuals with this perception of stuttering "are merely confessing that they have not read the recent literature" (p. 240).

However, when one considers stuttering from various points of view, for example, that of the professional, the audience, and the individual plagued with this disorder, one gets the impression that there is still much mystery and lack of understanding indeed. For instance, many professionals in the field of speech–language pathology still view this problem as an enigma. The audience may view stuttering as a disruption, and finally, the stutterer might think this problem is caused by a poltergeist (a mischievous ghost inside of them).

The mysteries surrounding stuttering are even more salient when one encounters the exceptionally severe stutterer. Some stutterers, by definition, have serious fluency disruptions in their speech, and, frequently, have a host of struggle mechanisms, troublesome histories, and evidence of complex causes.

The purposes of this chapter are to discuss and review a number of clinical issues that relate to exceptionally severe stutterers and to present in some detail how they can be diagnosed and treated.

Prior to our discussion of the nature and treatment of the exceptionally severe stutterer, we must establish our boundaries regarding certain aspects of the nature of stuttering, and attempt to further understand the disorder by defining the behaviors that we wish to examine and modify.

DEFINITION OF STUTTERING

The definition of stuttering provided here is not a revolutionary explanation of this centuries-old problem. It is, however, a conglomeration of other definitions (Brutten & Shoemaker, 1967; Wingate, 1964), along with our own considerations, to further synthesize the aspects of (1) what the stutterer does, (2) the effect of those behaviors on the individual, and (3) the impact of those behaviors on the environment. We offer the following definition:

> Stuttering is said to occur when the forward flow of speech with others is involuntarily disrupted by various motoric events, producing part-word repetitions and prolongations, either silent or audible, frequently accompanied by various accessory features, either simple or compound. These motoric disruptions, along with the accompanying accessory features, give the impression of struggle-type behaviors. There is frequently an alteration of appropriate rate and prosody, and often the individual experiences negative emotion during the speech disruption.[1]

[1]Our definition allows for only one kind of repetition, notably, part-word repetition. Ryan (1974) and Shine (1980) argue that whole-word repetitions should also be included as stutterings. Yet, information obtained during parental interviews (Johnson and associates, 1959) indicate an almost equal distribution of whole-word repetitions occurring between transitory and incipient stutterers. We favor including primarily those fluency-

It is essential, in this author's opinion, to consider the "involuntary disruption" in the forward flow of speech (Perkins, 1983). Wingate (1969) focused on disruption in speech flow in his simplified definition of stuttering as a "phonetic transition defect." He stated that "this should provide a valuable focus of orientation for both theoretic and therapeutic purposes." (p. 108) We comment later in this chapter on therapeutic purposes that may be served with this definition in mind.

The exceptionally severe stutterer typically manifests those characteristics that are identified as stuttering behaviors. Compared to typical stutterers, the severe stutterer displays: (1) greater frequency of stuttering in many if not most situations, (2) greater durations of stutterings, and (3) increased physical concomitants (greater struggle behaviors). These individuals appear to be more affected by their environments than typical stutterers. Many exceptionally severe stutterers tend to experience a reduction in the above characteristics in very relaxed situations, yet when their perceived stress raises slightly, they again experience severe symptoms. The mild and moderate stutterers report significant decreases in stuttering with decreased stress in their environments.

CHARACTERISTICS OF THE EXCEPTIONALLY SEVERE STUTTERER

The following are two examples from our files of individuals with exceptionally severe stuttering:

> William, 13 years old, with athetoid cerebral palsy, had rarely if ever talked in school. He wandered in the hallway, with extremely slow movements, almost always late for classes. He worked with his speech–langage pathologist for almost a year before he would attempt to talk with her. Once he did, in one-word units, it was apparent to her that he was an exceptionally severe stutterer. At the time of his evaluation for

---

disrupting characteristics that are unique to individuals who stutter thus eliminating whole-word repetitions from our definition. We recognize that some of these dysfluencies are often accompanied by an *abruptness of arrest* at the completion of each attempt on that word. Perhaps further clarification of this issue can come with detailed spectrographic analysis versus listener judgments. If it is indeed demonstrated that these whole-word repetitions are incomplete in their production, then they must be redefined as part-word repetitions. But, in the meantime, what does the clinician do? A good rule of thumb to follow is that if there is *any* doubt in the repetition with incompleteness of production, score that repetition as part-word.

admittance into our program, he demonstrated 75% stuttering in conversation, with a speaking rate of one-word-per-minute (WPM). He admitted that he had never been able to string a sentence together at one time. The following contributed to his overall rating on the Riley (1980) Stuttering Severity Instrument: 18 points for Frequency of stuttering (Reading, 80%; Job Task, 75%), 5 for Duration (10 sec), and a score of 10 on Physical Concomitants. His total score was 33, which yielded a classification of very severe.

Michael, 25 years old, was a clerk in a grocery store. His "assignment" was the "back door key." He would open the door for a delivery person, help unload the truck, and then sign for the merchandise received. He did not communicate verbally during these times. He was subsequently evaluated at a southern university, and in the report, the clinician stated that "it seems likely that there might be a neurological basis for some aspects of [Michael's] speech"and also that he was "the most severe stutterer I have ever encountered." When he attempted to speak, Michael's jaw made violent chewing movements, his arms and hands shook uncontrollably, and he demonstrated sporadic phonation. At the time of his evaluation for admittance into our program, he demonstrated 80% stuttering in conversation, with a speaking rate of 33 WPM. The following contributed to his overall rating on the Riley (1980) Stuttering Severity Instrument: Frequency of stuttering score of 18 (Reading, 50%; Job Task 80%), Duration score of 5 (20 seconds), and a score of 15 on Physical Concomitants. His total score was 38, which yielded a classification of very severe.

These two individuals present different problems, but they end up with the same classification. However, they are indeed different, and the approach to treatment will be influenced by these differences. We examine these two individuals later in this chapter by reporting their progress in therapy and how they are coping with long-term maintenance of new skills.

DISTRIBUTION OF STUTTERING SEVERITY IN THE GENERAL POPULATION

What percentage of the stuttering population are in the category of exceptionally (or very) severe stutterers? Soderberg (1962) sought to determine the "average" frequency of stuttering. When we reexamine these data, we find the following breakdown, using a modification of the Johnson, Darley, & Spriestersbach (1963) ratings:

Severity of Stuttering	% of Population
Mild	48
Moderate	17
Severe	25
Very severe	10

Thus, the very severe category accounts for only 10% of the stuttering population. If we were to combine the severe and very severe categories, these individuals would account for slightly over *one-third* of those who stutter. The data clearly demonstrate that the distribution of stuttering is skewed to the right and that approximately *two-thirds* of individuals who stutter fall into the mild and moderate categories. It is important to note that the above data from Soderberg reflect oral reading samples only, taken in a clinical setting.

Regardless of the question of the representativeness of these severities and the environment in which they were evoked, the fact remains that there is a relatively small subgroup of individuals who experience exceptionally severe suttering. This view is supported by other studies, such as Ryan (1980).

During the 4-year period of 1981-1984, a total of 135 individuals who stuttered were treated in the Summer Residence Stuttering Clinic (SRSC) held on the campus of the State University College of Arts and Science, Geneseo, New York. Enrollees participated in a 5-week, 200-hour, residential treatment program. The treatment consisted of a motoric reorientation of the speech mechanism, with emphasis on elimination of accessory features and the restoration of normal prosodic features, with slow-normal rates of speech.

The theoretical orientation and treatment program explained in this chapter are influenced heavily by the author's experience with stutterers seen in the SRSC. As will be seen, this group is atypical, primarily because it includes a high proportion of severe and very severe stutterers.

In the first place, minimum criterion for acceptance into this program is the presence of *moderate* stuttering, as measured on the Riley (1980) *Stuttering Severity Scale*. The population, therefore, is not a typical sample or an adequate cross-section of individuals who stutter, in that those who demonstrate less than moderate stuttering are excluded from this residential program. In other words, approximately 49% of those who

Table 4.1
Enrollments by Stuttering Severity in
the SRSC, 1981–1984

Severity	Number	Percent
Moderate	60	44.44
Severe	59	43.71
Very severe	16	11.85
	135	100.00

stutter (Soderberg, 1962) are not eligible for admittance into the SRSC program.

Table 4.1 shows the breakdown of enrollments in the SRSC by severity, over the past four summers (1981–1984). As can be seen, there is a near equal distribution of moderate and severe stutterers (44% each) with an additional 12% diagnosed as very severe.

These data, again, are not consistent with the distributions reported by Soderberg (1962) as typical of the stuttering population.

OTHER CHARACTERISTICS

Next, we examine additional characteristics of this group of 135 individuals who stutter: (1) gender, (2) familial incidence, and (3) handedness.

Examination of Table 4.2 reveals no significant differences between male and female stuttering as a function of the severity of their stutter-

Table 4.2
Severity versus Gender, Familial Incidence, and Handedness of 135 Enrollees
in the SRSC, 1981–1984

Severity	Gender[a]		Familial[b] Incidence		Handedness[c]	
	Male	Female	Yes	No	Right	Left
Moderate	88.8	11.7	73.3	26.7	90.0	10.0
Severe	86.4	13.6	64.4	35.6	86.4	13.6
Very severe	81.3	18.8	50.0	50.0	68.8	31.3
Means:	86.7	13.3	66.7	33.3	85.5	14.1

[a]$\chi^2(2) = .55$, n.s.
[b]$\chi^2(2) = 3.34$, n.s.
[c]$\chi^2(2) = 4.74$, n.s.

ing. Two-thirds of the stutterers in this population had a familial incidence of stuttering (parents, siblings, grandparents, and other blood relatives). It is interesting to note that family incidence of stuttering decreased with severity. The least severe group had the highest incidence. Kidd, Kidd, and Records (1978) reported familial incidence figures that were much lower (27% in one or both parents) in the stutterers they examined. They probed for only parental stuttering, but this difference still does not account for the much higher incidences reported among our group.

From Table 4.2, it is interesting to note that as the severity of stuttering increases, so does the incidence of left-handedness. As a matter of fact, left-handed individuals represent almost one-third of the very severe stutterers. The total group figures of approximately 86% right-handers and 14% left-handers are apparently different from distributions of handedness in the normal population. Hardyk, Goldman, and Petrinovich (1975) reported handedness in normal adults (males and females combined) as 90.4% right-handed and 9.6% left-handed.

Table 4.3, which compares familial incidence of stuttering and handedness of the 135 stutterers as a function of gender, reveals that approximately two-thirds of the males had incidence of familial stuttering, while females had only a 50% incidence. This is consistent with the results of Kidd et al. (1978), who also reported lower incidences of familial stuttering among females. Hardyk et al. (1975) reported normal males to be 89.5% right-handed and 10.5% left-handed; and females, 91.3% right-handed and 8.7% left-handed. In our data, the males who stuttered resemble the nonstuttering population in handedness, while the female stutterers have a much greater prominance toward left-handedness (61.1% right-handed vs. 38.9% left-handed) than does the nonstuttering female population.

Table 4.3
Gender versus Familial Incidence and Handedness in SRSC,
1981–1984.

Gender	Familial Incidence[a]		Handedness (%)[b]	
	Yes	No	Right	Left
Male	69.2	30.8	89.7	10.3
Female	50.0	50.0	61.1	38.9
Totals	66.7	33.3	85.9	14.1

[a]$\chi^2(1) = 1.80$, n.s.
[b]$\chi^2(1) = 8.34$, $p < .01$.

Table 4.4
Familial Incidence versus Handedness
in Enrollees in SRSC, 1981–1984

Familial Incidence	Handedness (%)[a]	
	Right	Left
Yes	88.9	11.1
No	80.0	20.0
Means	85.9	14.1

[a]$\chi^2(1) = 1.29$, n.s.

Table 4.4 compares handedness and familial incidence of the SRSC population. In this analysis, no statistically significant difference between the occurrence of stuttering in a family history and the handedness of the stutterer were present.

ATTITUDINAL MEASURES

Attitudinal measures are also considered in the admittance process to the SRSC program. Data have been collected, utilizing the S-24 Scale (Andrews & Cutler, 1974), which is a modification of the 36-item scale developed by Erickson (1969). Table 4.5 presents pre- and posttreatment scores for the 135 individuals enrolled over the 1981–1984 summers.

Andrews and Cutler (1974) found that their successfully treated stutterers obtained a mean score of 9 on their S-24 Scale, indicating that their treated group had attitudes about various aspects of communication that were consistent with nonstutterers (their nonstuttering controls scored a mean of 9.14). Examination of the data in Table 4.5 reveals that all of the SRSC groups had scores lower than 9, possibly indicating a "more healthy attitude" following treatment. Again, it must be kept in mind that the SRSC stuttering group is not "normally distributed" in severity, and quite possibly, gains made by these more severe stutterers were perceived by them to be more significant than might have occurred with a typical sample of stutterers. It is also interesting to note that the very severe group scored a bit higher (less positively) than the moderate and severe groups in both pre- and posttreatment scores, but not significantly so. Guitar (1976) points out that "pre-treatment factors are independent from pre-treatment stuttering measures," suggesting

Table 4.5
S-24 Scale[a] Values for Pre- and Posttreatment of 135 Enrollees
in the SRSC, 1981–1984

Severity	Number	Pretreatment	Posttreatment
Moderate	60	16.45	7.10
Male	53	16.90	7.60
Female	7	13.00	3.29
Severe	59	17.25	7.25
Male	51	17.37	7.20
Female	8	16.50	7.63
Very severe	16	17.69	8.31
Male	13	16.92	8.61
Female	3	21.00	7.00
Total	135	16.94	7.34
Male	117	16.71	7.44
Female	18	18.50	6.72

[a]Andrews and Cutler (1974).

that these attitudinal measures "tap an entirely different dimension of stuttering than do counts of stutters and syllables" (p. 598). Another way of stating the results of the above S-24 Scale measures is that less severe stutterers may still perceive the impact of their stuttering on the environment to be greater than the independent ratings of their severity by speech–language pathologists. This illustrates that an individual's perception of the impact of his/her stuttering on the environment may not correlate well with severity ratings.

Also, Table 4.5 reveals that the data for the 18 women (13.3% of the total treated) shows slight variations. The moderate female stutterers perceived less difficulty as reflected in the S-24 Scale for pretreatment than did moderate male stutterers, but the severe and very severe females rated themselves higher than did their male counterparts. Examination of Table 4.5 reveals that the S-24 scale scores increase among both groups (male and female) as severity increases.

Silverman and Zimmer (1979) found that female stutterers evidenced a higher level of self-esteem than their male stuttering counterparts. This appears to be the case in the posttreatment scores presented for the moderate and very severe groups of female stutterers. The severe group scored slightly higher than their male stuttering counterparts. (A much more in-depth examination of the problem of women who stutter can be found in Silverman, Chapter 3, this volume).

SPEECH RATE AND PROSODY

The case studies presented earlier, William and Michael, illustrate the importance of speech rate in the exceptionally severe stutterer. William and Michael obtained the same severity ratings (very severe) prior to treatment. The most obvious difference was their rates of speech prior to treatment. Even though neither would fall within the normal range, William's speech was certainly more debilitating to him in conversation with others. William's response was not to speak, whereas Michael uttered gutteral sounds consistently unitl a word finally came out. The *rate of speech* should be a consideration in the pretreatment evaluation of the stutterer, as there is certainly a large difference between William and Michael (1 WPM versus 33 WPM). There is also a big difference between the stutterer who demonstrates broken words and pacing, with a basic monotone, from the stutterer with much more normal prosodic features, such as better speech flow with more appropriate inflection. Obviously, rate and prosody differences in severe stutterers such as in the above two cases must be dealt with in treatement.

DIAGNOSTIC CONSIDERATIONS

We typically evaluate the extent and severity of stuttering through the examination of its frequency, duration, and physical concomitants. However, other factors may need to be taken into consideration. Martin and Haroldson (1981) hypothesized that "the environment of the speech interruption, and the experiences of the observer" may need to be taken into account in the evaluational process (p. 62). These additional factors are extremely difficult to measure in a diagnostic evaluation. Guitar (1976) also includes pretreatment attitudes, stuttering behaviors, and personality measures.

Obviously, as professionals we have an obligation to our clients to provide them with as complete an evaluation as possible, identifying those aspects of the stutterer's behaviors that need to be modified through treatment. We need to assess attitudes and behavioral patterns of the environment that either encourage or discourage fluency of speech, and finally, we need to take into consideration the feelings and attitudes of the person who stutters.

How does one judge factors to determine severity of stuttering? Various measurements of stuttering severity have been reported by listeners. Lewis and Sherman (1951) and Naylor (1953) attempted to measure the consistency of judgments of severity. Utilizing a 9-point interval rating scale, they determined that their listeners could rank stuttering severity solely on the basis of audio samples of stuttering. Cullinan, Prather, and Williams (1963) employed various interval-scaling techniques, as well as direct magnitude estimation (DME), and found little differences in their results. However, they found that DME interjudge reliability was lower than any of the other interval scaling measures. Schiavetti, Sacco, Metz, and Sitler (1983) demonstrated that DME measures, rather than interval scaling measures, were more accurate in scaling severity of stuttering through listening tasks.

Scales developed by Johnson et al. (1963) and Riley (1972, 1980) deal with the following dimensions: (1) frequency of stuttering, (2) duration of stuttering, and (3) physical concomitants. These are important stuttering characteristics to measure. We recommend adding two additional dimensions to the diagnostic evaluation: rate of speech (measured with and without stutterings and pauses) and prosodic features.

Reviewing these five dimensions shows that the first two are the easiest to assess. One can transcribe a recorded sample of speech and assess both the frequency and the duration of stuttering. It is recommended that both reading and conversational samples be obtained and analyzed. Subjective judgments of the presence and extent of physical concomitants are more difficult to make, but can be done using the Riley (1980) scale.

Currently, there are no rate scales to apply regarding the range of various severities of stuttering and accompanying rates of speech. According to Darley (1940), in his examination of 200 normal speakers, normal oral-reading rates range from 129 to 222 WPM, with a mean rate of 148 WPM. Certainly the speech–language pathologist should attempt to establish speaking rates above 129 WPM in successfully treated stutterers, except in cases that present additional mitigating factors.

The final dimension, prosody, is an important consideration in the flow of speech. For example, if an individual speaks in a monotone, the audience might react with "that's a dull speaker" or "boring to listen to." Perkins (1973) provided goals for generalizing normal speech in stuttering treatment and specifically refers to a goal for establishing normal prosody. Treatment modes that advocate a normal flow of speech without regard to more normal prosodic features tend to produce speakers that fall into that "dubious fluency level" discussed by Adams and Runyan (1981). One technique for establishing more normal prosody is discussed later in this chapter under the heading of "Highlighting."

TREATMENT RATIONALE

Andrews, Guitar, and Howie (1980) assessed the "state of the art" in stuttering treatment and described the effects of various modes of treatment through meta-analysis (a way of synthesizing different treatments under common treatment effects). Their findings indicated the following "most effective forms of therapy": (1) prolonged speech, (2) gentle onset techniques, and (3) rhythm. Speech therapy, utilizing prolonged speech (Andrews & Tanner, 1982; Boberg, 1976; Healy & Adams, 1981; Ingham & Packman, 1977; and Resnick, Wendiffensen, Ames, & Meyer, 1978) has proven to be an effective means of altering stuttering behaviors. Gentle onset and air flow techniques have also been reported with positive results (Andrews & Tanner, 1982). Miller (1982) stated, "It appears reasonable to conclude that airflow therapy, in its various forms, provides a measure of aid . . . . The average stutterer in an airflow therapy program will probably experience a sizable reduction in stuttering" (pp. 197–198). Fluency-shaping techniques provide good results as reported by Blaesing (1982), Mallard & Kelly (1982), and Webster (1974). This approach typically involves the following: (1) full breath, (2) gentle onset techniques, and (3) syllable transitions. The application of these combined techniques allows the stutterer to work in a more integrated manner in modifying his/her stuttering behaviors. An additional benefit of this treatment approach is the emphasis the above researchers have placed on transfer techniques, practice suggestions, and specific goals (most notably Webster, 1974).

In summary, we advocate an integrated approach to the treatment of the exceptionally severe stutterer. By combining techniques such as air flow, prolonged speech, and gentle onset, we have designed an integrated program to assist the exceptionally severe stutterer in new fluency skills. The heaviest influence in our treatment regimes comes from Van Riper (1973). We have attempted to modify his suggestions for treatment, using very specific, individualized objectives throughout our treatment program. We offer the following outline of treatment strategies, which we have found to be very useful and successful in the SRSC Program.

Treatment in the SRSC

At the outset, it must be stated that we address the problems of the exceptionally severe stuterers. We operationally define our program as the GEMS Program, which consists of:

G—General explanation of the overall treatment program
E—Exposure of stuttering and symptomology
M—Modification of stuttering and new techniques promo-
   ting fluency
S—Stabilization and transfer

General Explanation

We have found it beneficial for the very severe stutterer to be provided
with a comprehensive overview of all the aspects of treatment prior to
its initiation. This tends to remove the mystery of what we are going to
do in the treatment program. As each objective in the program is completed, the individual is more likely to perceive how that objective fits
into the treatment process.

Exposure of Stuttering

As noted earlier, a high priority is given in the SRSC Program to elimination of accessory features. It has been our experience that once these
accessory features have been identified and eliminated, the stutterer will
experience, in most instances, "easier" stuttering.

As part of the exposure stage, we immediately address accessory features that interfere with the stutterer's concentration on the production
of the speech mechanism. Semour, Ruggiero, and McEneany (1983) re-
marked on the importance of these accessory features: "The clinical
evaluation of stuttering needs to include visual as well as auditory stuttering behavior . . . . To ignore the nonverbal aspects of stuttering is to
ignore a vital aspect of the disorder" (pp. 219–220). Eye contact, for example, plays an extremely important role in listener reactions to stuttering. Tachell, VanDen Berg, & Lehrman (1983) reported that the
frequency of a speaker's eye contact was more strongly related to listeners' perceptions than fluency.

We recommend the following as a check-list of accessory features:

1. gross movements of the body (including arms and legs, hands,
head, shoulders, and general postural changes);
2. finer movements of the body (including eye movements, eye contact, eyeblinks, eyebrow movement, nostril flaring, facial twitching, and
tongue protrusions);
3. breath stream/laryngeal (including talking on "residual air," sudden inhalations or vocalizations on inhalations, pitch changes or pitch
hikes, and decreasing or increasing volume);

4. verbal accessories (such as starters, retrials, circumlocutions, and sound substitutions or additions).

An alternate check list is provided by Peins (1984, pp. 118–121).

To eliminate accessory features, we utilize a technique referred to as implosion therapy. This technique is different from the more familiar systematic desensitization. Kanfer & Goldstein (1975), in their discussion of systematic desensitization, state that it has as a basic assumption "a fear response can be inhibited by substituting an activity which is antagonistic to the fear response. Desensitization is accomplished by gradually exposing an individual in small steps to the feared situation while he is performing the activity that is antagonistic to anxiety" (p. 230). Rather than utilize systematic desensitization (which is a process that occurs over a relatively long period of time), we prefer to use implosive therapy to facilitiate the elimination of accessory features (Adams, 1982; Van Riper, 1973). Kanfer and Goldstein (1975) explain that the purpose of implosive therapy is to "produce a frightening experience in the person of such magnitude that [it] will actually *lessen* the fear of the particular situation rather than heighten it" (p. 257). Gendelman (1977) lists four steps in her confrontation of the aspects of the client's fears of stuttering that are similar to implosive therapy for accessory features.

Implosive therapy helps the stutterer to confront and eliminate accessory features in a more rapid fashion than systematic desensitization. We have been very successful in the sudden, short-term elimination of these features. We have advocated that this implosive therapy be done both in clinical and outpatient settings. With this approach, the stutterer not only quickly learns to eliminate accessory features, but has the opportunity to assess the impact that these behaviors have had on his/her speech. This elimination of accessory features also tends to generate an "immediate positive change" in treatment. Thus, the implosion technique provides "positive worth" to the client in the initial stages of treatment.

The last consideration in the exposure stage is the examination of the motoric events related to the moment of stuttering. We approach this in the following order:

1. Prestuttering events (anticipation of stuttering, tensions, accessories/starters, breathing patterns, eye contact, emotions, and preformations (preparatory sets).
2. Poststuttering events (tensions in the mechanism, breathing patterns, eye contact, emotions, and posture changes).
3. During-stuttering events (air/sound flow, tensions and tremors in

the mechanism, eye-contact, type of stuttering, voicing appropriateness, hard contacts, focal point of articulation, accessory features, and lact of movement).

A careful examination of these events informs the stutterer of what processes of speech were produced correctly and where errors of that process occurred. It is those errors of the process that are modified by the individual in the following phase of the treatment.

Modification of Stuttering

It is at this stage that the stutterer practices carefully controlled movements that allow him/her to continue the forward flow of speech (the antithesis of the "phonetic transition defect" concept introduced by Wingate (1969). This allows the stutterer to feel the forward flow (with slightly reduced rates in a monotonous tone). The main goal is not to strive for slow-sounding speech, but rather to make initiating and transitional movements in such a way that the individual "feels" what the articulators are doing in this process. We refer to this feel of positioning and movement as *proprioceptive awareness* of what the mechanism is doing while moving forward. We stress that the individual "not listen to *how* it sounds"; rather, the person is instructed to *feel the forward flow and continuity of movement* that he/she is *voluntarily* initiating and maintaining. At this point in the treatment process, we again repudiate Wingate's (1969) notion of "stuttering as a phonetic transition defect" and explain that it is the *voluntary* movements initiated by the stutterer that overcomes the stuttering (which is involuntary).

We practice this process in the following manner:

1. reduced rates with monosyllabic word units;
2. reduced rates with polysyllabic word units;
3. reduced rates with short phrases spoken as one word, with continuous flow (not continuous *voicing*).

We define the above short phrases as a *breath flow*, that is, speech that can be spoken in one normal intake of air. The stutterer is encouraged to speak in several short phrases, than take a breath, and then continue the process. Of course, it is also stressed that these "breathing breaks" be brief in nature and occur at appropriate junctures in a sentence.

Stabilization and Transfer

The last process in treatment encourages the stutterer to practice variations in rate and to begin to add elements of normal prosodic features. The rule of thumb to be followed is that at low-normal rates of speech, the individual must add appropriate prosodic features. Many observers in our program have described such speech as deliberate rather than slow with the application of good prosody. Variations of inflection, for example, have the effect of "masking" slower rates. Perkins (1973) pointed out, "Much of the objection to slow rates turns out to be in reality objection to monotony. Expressive speech at slow-normal rates has been proven to be reasonably acceptable" (p. 288).

At this point, many stutterers encounter an important difficulty. Their speech attempts match target behaviors outlined for them, while in the clinical setting, where there tends to be very little pressure and stress. Nevertheless, when they begin to transfer these new skills out of the clinical setting, they typically report difficulties in performance. Prior to exposing our stutterers to outside situations for this type of skill application, we find it advantageous to teach them to examine their levels of stress. Stress awareness and reduction can have a positive effect on the speech process. One explanation for this beneficial effect was advanced by Zimmerman (1980), who stated "lowering stress in speaking situations may serve to reduce dysfluency by lowering gains of reflex pathways and/or reduce movement variability" (p. 133–134).

Schwartz (1976) presented an interesting discussion of the stutterer's seven basic stressors. We have modified this list of seven stressors into the following major and minor categories: Major stressors include (1) speed stress, (2) word or sound stress, (3) authority figure stress, and (4) situational stress. Minor stressors include (5) stress of uncertainty, (6) physical stress, and (7) external stress. This major and minor dichotomy applies to most stutterers but may not be appropriate for all of them. For example, a recent graduate of our program informed us that the "minor stress of uncertainty appeared to be his greatest stress. Certainly, regularly scheduled reexamination of these stressors relative to their importance with the individual is recommended following treatment.

It is common to hear a stutterer state, "When I talk to _____, I do well, but when _____ enters the room, I fall apart," or "Why is it that when I go into *that* store, I have so much trouble?" Another of our recent graduates reported to us that his speech skills were excellent on the job, on the telephone, and while talking to his parents, but when he casually spoke to his friends, he experienced some stuttering. In order to deal with such difficulties, we offer the following suggestion in the treatment process. *We recommend that the individual vary the speed of his/her speech, commensurate with the level of stress that he/she is perceiving, in order to maintain the fluent, forward flow of speech.* The concept of GEARS (*G*o *E*asily and *A*djust your *R*eactions) is introduced at this point. We discuss "gearing up" (making faster movements) and "gearing down" (making slower movements). As stress *increases*, the stutterer should gear down to a more comfortable rate, in order to keep the forward flow of speech. When stress *decreases*, the stutterer can gear up acordingly. The rule of thumb to follow here is that when the individual gears up or down he/she must maintain that preselected rate throughout that breath flow. Then, after an additional breath (following that breath phrase), the individual can select the next "appropriate gear." Speeding up or slowing down through a particular breath phrase does not sound natural.

In order for the stutterer to be specific about levels of stress, it is necessary to rank *heirarchies of stress* under each of the stress categories. The individual lists the most threatening condition as Number 1 and the "least threatening" as Number 10. Thus, a typical heirarchy of authority figure stress might be (1) boss, (2) strangers, (3) parents, (4) grandparents, (5) casual friends, (6) close friends, (7) spouse, (8) brother/sister, (9) child, and (10) animal or pet. These stress analyses should be customized for each stutterer, and, ultimately, stutterers should rank them under their own major and minor categories. Again, periodic review of the import and ranking of subcategories of stress should be undertaken.

Coupling the concepts of stressors and GEARS, the individual is prepared to handle his/her speech in a more positive fashion and in more settings outside of the clinical environment.

Finally, we practice the integration of motor control and motor planning in a total process. Rather than focus on the anticipation of the moment of stuttering, we practice rate variations, incorporating good inflectional patterns with slow-normal rates. Wendell and Cole (1961) suggested that "a therapy program with stutterers must consider speech as a whole and that it is not sufficient to work toward the goal of modifying the 'stuttering block' " (p. 286).

We approach this goal of integration of the smooth flow of speech through a technique we call *highlighting*. This affords the integration of the techniques taught and the facilitation of more normal-sounding speech. This technique is so-named because when one wants to call attention to certain items on the printed page, one takes a colored marker and runs ink over the line. The marker highlights that line, but the color is transparent and does not truly distort the integrity of the printed page.

A graphic example of highlighting would be "This is the way to achieve good highlighting in speech."The individual adds slightly rising inflections to each underscored sound (or sound combination). This is done very slightly so as not to disturb the continuity of flow. The individual can slightly reduce the speed of each of these transitions, adding slight rising iflection at each accentuated sound. Loudness control should be consistent throughout the utterance. It may be said that each of the underscored sounds are emphasized, but if the stutterer also correctly monitors rate and inflection, the resulting speech sounds quite natural.

Once stabilization has occurred in the clinical setting, the individual is ready to transfer activities out into the environment. A great deal of practice in these outside communication situations is necessary. We provide the client with detailed evaluational forms for these situations, and he/she tape-records them for later detailed analysis. Some situations require groups of stutterers, with or without the clinician present, and others require stutterers be alone. As all of these conversation situations are tape-recorded, the stutterer can compare the effects of audience size in these situations on his/her attempts at transfer. There is a great deal of role-playing practiced in the clinical setting as well, assessing the effects of varying stress and noting adjustments and reactions on the part of the stutterer. Utilization of a video-tape recorder at this stage is extremely beneficial to the client.

Transfer of skills back into the home environment is the next order of business. Each client develops, with the assistance of the clinical staff, a customized maintenance program, based on the strengths and weaknesses perceived not only by the stutterer but also by the entire clinical staff. We thus do not advocate a "cookbook" maintenance program, but one that is custom-tailored to best suit the needs of each individual treated in the program.

As the individual may return to the Center for reevaluation at appropriate intervals, these custom-designed maintanance strategies, such as review of overall skills and daily or weekly assessments of difficult sounds or situations, are discussed and altered to meet the new needs of the individual.

As far as appropriate rates of speech are concerned, we do not advocate rates that are measured at less than 100 WPM. We advocate the teaching of a variable rate of 120–150 WPM, which is a comfortable listening rate for the audience. However, with those individuals who demonstrate obvious and particularly severe physical involvements, *any* improvement in the forward flow of speech is likely to have a positive impact on that individual's environment. Returning to the case presented earlier, William achieved a 40 WPM rate at the termination of treatment (up from 1 WPM pretreatment). His measured stuttering at the end of the program was reduced to 3% (from 75% pretreatment). One year later, in a follow-up session, William's rate was measured at 33 WPM, with 3% stuttering. Is William a failure? Yes, since he failed to achieve rates within normal limits for speech, and no, since he maintained his new skills at posttreatment levels of stuttering frequency for well over a year. His speaking rate dropped slightly, but he reported significant improvements in himself and his effect on his environment.

Michael, 3 years following treatment, still takes a long time to get his point across to his listeners. However, he does not flail his arms and hands as he did prior to treatment. His current rate of speech ranges from 60 to 80 WPM (33 WPM before treatment and 90 WPM immediately following treatment). His level of stuttering at the end of the treatment program was 2% and at the present time is 5–10% (pretreatment frequency was 75%). He is now working for a local power company in the mailroom (a talking job), and he has started a local self-help group for stutterers in his city. He had a T-shirt made up and wears it around the city. It says "Please talk to me—I need the practice."

COMMITMENT TO TREATMENT

How much commitment must the stutterer (and treatment staff) make to achieving the goal of fluency? Robert Owens, one of our colleagues, has on his office wall a hanging that says:

Communication training without the environment is like toilet training without the potty.

Those who attempt to treat the stutterer by introducing new techniques in the clinical setting without establishing them into real-life situations are forgetting the potty. In order to illustrate this point, let us look at a possible alternative we use to enlarge the scope of treatment.

THE TRIAD OF TREATMENT

Rehabilitation can be said to involve three main foci: (1) technique; (2) life-style adjustments, and (3) self-esteem. The following example serves to integrate these three aspects of treatment.

A problem very near and dear to most people is the problem of excess weight. Most individuals who suffer from this problem (including this author) have struggled through many different weight reduction programs. An individual can participate in a *technique* of an organized weight-reduction program or can attempt self-treatment. Once the desired goal has been reached, one of two things will happen. He/she will either maintain the weight loss (usually with some slight regression) or regress to the point of gaining back most, if not more, weight than before. What determines the course a person might take? Several factors seem to be important here. First, the person must make certain *life-style adjustments* following the successful tratment. For example, new, tighter-fitting clothing in a smaller size could purchased, and the old, baggier clothes discarded. This would be one important way to reduce the temptation of regaining the weight, that is, to avoid having clothes to fall back on if the weight is regained! If there is weight gain, then a decision must be made to lose it, or it will be necessary to buy new, larger clothes! Also, new eating patterns that have been learned must be reinforced as regular behaviors to be maintained. The person may be introduced to new environments, such as the beach (with a new bathing suit). The key, controlling factor of these life-style adjustments is self-esteem, or how the person feels about him/herself. To maintain rehabilitative gains, self-esteem must remain high; the person must seek out reinforcements from the environment initially but in the final analysis, must find that reinforcement from within. After a person has gone through a weight-loss program, and others notice the wight loss, their initial comments might be "Wow, you look great!" Soon, however, others no longer comment on how good one looks, and it is up to the individual who has lost the weight to reinforce him/herself on appearance, and other benefits. If that individual does not engage in self-reinforcement, then the weight-maintenance program will surely suffer, with a resultant loss in self-esteem and the abandonment of the new, limiting dietary pattern necessary for weight loss maintenance. Regression is likely to follow, with weight gain possibly approaching pre–weight-loss conditions. The individual is often initially successful in losing the desired weight but is not successful in maintaining that weight loss.

Two ways of encouraging maintenance of weight loss are (1) making good life-style adjustments (and adhering to them), and (2) increasing one's self-esteem. As long as an individual feels good about changes he/she has made, those changes are likely to be maintained. This triad of treatment is essential in the transfer and successful long-term use of skills, and should be stressed in stuttering treatment programs.

Owen (1981) provided us with excellent guidelines for the generalization and maintenance of skills over a long-term basis. These include

1. personal goal setting and planning;
2. self-observation, self-monitoring, and self-recording;
3. modifying environments, setting events, controlling stimuli that elicit the behaviors to be maintained;
4. self-administered reinforcement and adverse consequences;
5. covert strategies, including self-instruction and imagery techniques;
6. other adjuncts that will increase personal resilience. (p. 38)

At the same time, clinicians must be sensitive to reasons for failure. Perkins (1979) suggested four types of stutterers who may be likely to fail: (1) those who try hard but fail, (2) those who understand the techniques but cannot apply them, (3) those who profess a desire to sound normal but too easily lose control, and (4) those who have mastered skills yet prefer to stutter. We offer a fifth reason for failure: (5) those who work "part-time" on skill application.

Behaviorists who treat stuttering explain that if an individual regresses, then he/she should be "recycled" through entire treatment programs. This implies that someone has not done the job adequately. If the speech–language pathologist does not deal with some aspect of what motivates that individual, or how he/she reacts in certain situations, then further treatment is limited to the recycling of the laboratory technique. Of course, those who advocate such techniques make the assumption that the newly gained skills become automatic upon successful treatment. Oh, if that were so! It would then be a simple matter to "mass teach" these techniques to all speech–language pathologists, the problem of stuttering would soon be eliminated, and we would eliminate the need for books such as this one! The only mass teaching we have discovered is in the inappropriate application of the same type of program to those who are exceptionally severe stutterers. Given our current state-of-the-art in stuttering treatment, no such paradigm has emerged, despite the claims of some regarding their rates of success. The point being made here is that recycling is inadequate in dealing with regression with exceptionally severe stutterers. Instead, these individuals need to consider reactions to the environment as well as their own motivation in applying techniques on a regular, disciplined basis in order to maintain newly gained fluency skills.

Owen (1981) compared results of treatment in various programs, such as cigarette and alcohol rehabilitiation, and, following a 3-month period, the abstainers averaged about 40%. At 12 months, the abstainers were between 25 and 30%. How can we assure higher, long-term success rates with these types of problems, and also with stuttering rehabilitation? The answer, we believe, lies in the perception of *value* that the individual places on new speech skills. Also, group support, in the form of groups for parents or significant others, or self-help groups is necessary in order to provide external motivation and support in maintaining skills.

In the initial stages following stuttering treatment, the individual usually is bombarded with praise from the environment. When he/she demonstrates new speech that has eliminated the stuttering behaviors, people all around are typically amazed and pleased. In fact, this may lead to regression in the individual who has just undergone treatment.

The stutterer may begin to perform only for the environment, which has recently provided the positive reinforcement for good speech. This performance at selected times will occur in order to draw praise, but the individual may be more likely to lapse back into old speaking habits when that praise is later not provided. The stutterer then is working part time on skill application, working only during times that the environment is reinforcing. This indicates the lack of self-evaluation and self-esteem in doing a good job first of all for oneself, rather than for the environment. Accomplishing the former will simultaneously accomplish the latter.

Must the exceptionally severe stutterer make a *commitment* to him/herself rather than a *contribution* to the environment? The following anecdote (author unknown) may more accurately clarify the question:

> A chicken and a pig were walking down the street and happened by a restaurant, which had a sign in the window: "Ham and Egg Special Today." The chicken said to the pig, "Let's go in and have breakfast!" The pig replied to the chicken, "Wait a minute. An egg from you is a *contribution*, but ham from me is a real *commitment!*

The stutterer, who like the chicken, makes his/her contribution only when the environment demands new skill application, does not take a total, integrated approach to altering stuttering in familiar as well as new speaking environments (such as where there is no praise for new skill application). The stutterer may then revert back to old speech skills, demonstrating stuttering. The stutterer who is apt to be successful in using new skills in most, if not all, situations is more like the pig, making a real commitment. The speech–language pathologist, we believe, has the responsibility of instilling this concept in the stutterer very early in the therapeutic process.

DISMISSAL FROM FORMAL TREATMENT

At what point is the exceptionally severe stutterer ready for dismissal from formal treatment? Adams and Runyan (1981) raised a cogent issue when they stated, "we believe that the stutterer who is most ready for release from rehabilitation and who is likely to maintain his(her) improvement is the patient whose speech is objectively and perceptually indistinguishable from normal" (p. 215). Nevertheless, they also caution against releasing rehabilitated stutterers whose speech is free from stuttering, yet do not sound natural. They describe clients such as these as having "dubious fluency." We feel that these clients lack rates and pro-

Table 4.6
Treatment Results, by Severity Ratings (pretreatment) for Enrollees
in SRSC, 1981–1984 (Percent of Words Stuttered)

Dimension	Moderate	Severe	Very severe
Pretreatment	13.85	20.15	43.75
Posttreatment	.26	.37	.69

sodic features within normal limits. Wingate (1976) explains: "Funda-
mentally, speech is an undulating vocalized sound, a more-or-less
continuous tone that evidences substantial changes in its various aspects
while being produced. Within certain qualifications, these changes are
referred to as the prosody of speech" (p. 259).

Stuttering treatment programs usually state dismissal criteria such as
a certain percentage of stuttering (or fluency) as a condition of release
from treatment. We certainly do not disagree with this procedure, but
when one is faced with the reality of the exceptionally severe stutterer,
variations in rigid criteria are certainly in order. For instance, if the exceptionally severe stutterer achieves 95% fluency, that certainly is a reasonable criterion for dismissal. However, if that level of fluency is 70%,
and the individual demonstrated only 30% prior to treatment, the 70%
fluency level might indeed be acceptable for dismissal. Also, if that individual has learned to master good prosodic features, and uses effective rate manipulation, the residual stuttering artifacts may not
significantly influence his/her successes in the environment.

Table 4.6 examines pre- and posttreatment percentages of stuttering
for all three severity groups of the 135 stutterers enrolled in the SRSC
over a 4-year period. Prior to treatment, the very severe group presented
more than twice the stuttering of the severe group and over three times
that of the moderate group. Both the moderate and severe groups
achieved below .005% words stuttered following treatment, while the
very severe group (12% of those enrolled) still achieved less than 1%
stuttering following treatment. Although these results demonstrate excellent improvements following intensive treatment, they do point out
that not everyone comes away with the same gains.

TREATMENT SUMMARY

What have we advocated regarding the treatment of the exceptionally
severe stutterer? We have recommended a direct attack on their unique
pattern of accessory features. Following this, we advocate the examination of sound production and knowledge of the speech production

mechanism. As that is accomplished, we advocate the examination, in detail, of the stuttering itself, and we introduce motoric modifications to effectively maintain the forward flow of speech on a voluntary basis. We also suggest an awareness and assessment of stress in the environment and the application of a rate-variation methodology in skill application. We advocate that the speech–language clinician provide motivation to the client, at the outset of treatment, regarding self-evaluation and self-reinforcement skills. Certainly, criteria need to be set regarding dismissal; however, the decision when to dismiss must be based on the extent of the stutterer's problems, as well as other factors, such as accompanying physical limitations.

Of course, we advocate intensive treatment for the individual with an exceptionally severe stuttering problem. Unfortunately, intensive, residential programs are not commonplace at the time of this writing. However, they need not hamper the scheduling of this type of client *as often as possible.*

TRAINING PERSPECTIVES

When is one adequately trained to work with individuals who stutter? This question is certainly a difficult one to answer. When the speech–language clinician completes formal academic training, he/she typically has taken a course at the undergraduate or graduate level in fluency disorders and has participated in at least 25 hours of supervised practicum in fluency disorders. Certainly, additional training beyond this point is necessary. Speech–language pathologists who have a sincere desire to work with individuals who stutter need to be motivated to expand their knowledge of stuttering through participation in additional coursework, attendence in workshops and short courses on the nature and treatment of fluency disorders, and other related continuing education experiences. The expansion of training must not only include increased understanding of the problem, but should also include an increased understanding of the person who stutters and all the difficulties he/she encounters on a daily basis because of that stuttering.

The speech–language pathologist might be somewhat hesitant in scheduling an individual who demonstrates severe symptoms of stuttering. If so, it would be wise to examine one's own feelings and attitudes toward stuttering in order to identify those factors that might impede effectiveness. An excellent self-efficacy scale has been presented by Rudolph, Manning, and Sewell (1983), and readers are referred to this source. Once the clinician can identify those aspects of stuttering therapy about which he/she lacks confidence or skill, and then takes action to improve in those areas, he/she will no doubt be more effective with this population.

When the speech–language clinician is confronted by an exceptionally severe stutterer, that clinician must rank the priorities of each phase of the stutterer's problem and design an approach that will generate both short- and long-term success. There is no greater feeling of success than when the clinician hears an exceptionally severe stutterer say to his mother at the end of his successful treatment: "This is the one gift I have been saving—all of my life—to be able to talk like this!"

REFERENCES

Adams, M. R. (1982). A case report on the use of flooding in stuttering therapy. *Journal of Fluency Disorders, 7*, 343–354.

Adams, M. R. & Runyan, C. M. (1981). Stuttering and fluency: Exclusive events or points on a continuum? *Journal of Fluency Disorders, 6*, 197–218.

Andrews, G., Craig, A., Feyer, A., Hoddinott, S., Howie, P., & Neilson, M. (1983). Stuttering: A review of research findings and theories circa 1982. *Journal of Speech and Hearing Disorders, 48*, 226–245.

Andrews, G., & Cutler, J. (1974). Stuttering therapy: The relation between changes in symptom level and attitudes. *Journal of Speech and Hearing Disorders, 39*, 312–319.

Andrews, G., Guitar, B., & Howie, P. (1980). Meta-analysis of the effects of stuttering treatment. *Journal of Speech and Hearing Disorders, 45*, 287–307.

Andrews, G. and Tanner, S. (1982). Stuttering: The results of 5 days treatment with an airflow technique. *Journal of Speech and Hearing Disorders, 47*, 427–429.

Blaesing, L. (1982). A multidisciplinary approach to individualized treatment of stuttering. *Journal of Fluency Disorders, 7*, 203–218.

Bloodstein, O. (1981). *A handbook on stuttering* (3rd ed.). Chicago: National Easter Seal Society.

Boberg, E. (1976). Intensive group therapy program for stutterers. *Human Communication, 1*, 29–42.

Brutten, E. J., and Shoemaker, D. J. (1967). *The modification of stuttering.* Englewood Cliffs, NJ: Prentice-Hall, Inc.

Cullinan, W. L., Prather, E. M., & Williams, D. E. (1963). Comparisons of procedures for scaling severity of stuttering. *Journal of Speech and Hearing Research, 2*, 187–194.

Darley, F. L. (1940). *A normative study of oral reading rate.* Unpublished master's thesis, University of Iowa.

Erickson, R. L. (1969). Assessing communication attitudes among stutterers. *Journal of Speech and Hearing Research, 12*, 711–724.

Gendleman, E. G. (1977). Confrontation in the treatment of stuttering. *Journal of Speech and Hearing Disorders, 42*, 85–89.

Guitar, B. (1976). Pretreatment factors associated with the outcome of stuttering therapy. *Journal of Speech and Hearing Research, 19*, 590–600.

Hardyck, C., Goldman, R., & Petrinovich, L. (1975). Handedness and sex and race and age. *Human Biology, 3*, 369–375.

Healey, E. C., & Adams, M. R. (1981). Rate reduction strategies used by normally fluent and stuttering children and adults. *Journal of Fluency Disorders, 6,* 1–14.

Ingham, R. J., & Packman, A. (1977). Treatment and generalization effects in an experimental treatment for a stutterer using contingency management and speech rate control. *Journal of Speech and Hearing Disorders, 42,* 394–407.

Johnson, W., and associates. (1959). *The onset of stuttering.* Minneapolis: University of Minnesota Press.

Johnson, W., Darley, F., & Spriestersbach, D. (1963). *Diagnostic methods in speech pathology.* New York: Harper and Row.

Kanfer, F., & Goldstein, A., (1975). *Helping people change.* New York: Pergammon.

Kidd, K., Kidd, J., and Records, M. (1978). The possible cause of the sex ratio in stuttering and its implications. *Journal of Fluency Disorders, 3,* 13–23.

Lewis, D., & Sherman, D. (1951). Measuring the severity of stuttering. *Journal of Speech and Hearing Disorders, 16,* 320–326.

Mallard, A. R., & Kelly, J. S. (1982). The precision fluency shaping program: Replication and evaluation. *Journal of Fluency Disorders, 7,* 287–294.

MIller, S. (1982). Airflow therapy programs: Fact and/or fiction. *Journal of Fluency Disorders, 7,* 187–202.

Naylor, R. V. (1953). A comparative study of methods of estimating the severity of stuttering. *Journal of Speech and Hearing Disorders, 18,* 30–37.

Owen, N. (1981). Facilitating maintenance of behavior change. In E. Boberg (Ed.) *Maintenance of fluency.* New York: Elsevier.

Peins, M. (Ed.) (1984). *Contemporary approaches in stuttering therapy.* Boston: Little, Brown and Company.

Perkins, W. H. (1973). Replacement of stuttering with normal speech. 1. rationale. *Journal of Speech and Hearing Disorders, 38,* 283–294.

Perkins, W. H. (1979). From psychoanalysis to discoordination. In H. Gregory (Ed.), *Controversies about stuttering therapy.* Baltimore: University Park Press.

Perkins, W. H. (1983). The problem of definition: Commentary on 'stuttering'. *Journal of Speech and Hearing Disorders, 48,* 246–248.

Resnick, P., Wendiggensen, R., Ames, S., & Meyer, V. (1978). Systematic slowed speech: A new treatment in stuttering. *Behavioral Research and Therapy, 16,* 161–167.

Riley, G. (1972). A stuttering severity instrument for children and adults. *Journal of Speech and Hearing Disorders, 37,* 314–322.

Riley, G. (1980). Stuttering severity instrument for children and adults. (rev. ed.) Tigard, Or: C. C. Publications.

Rudolph, S. R., Maning, W. H., & Sewell, W. R. (1983). The use of self-efficacy scaling in training student clinicians: implications for working with stutterers. *Journal of Fluency Disorders, 8,* 55–75.

Ryan, B. (1974). *Programmed therapy for stuttering in children and adults.* Springfield, IL: Thomas.

Ryan, B. (1980). Maintenance programs in progress. In E. Boberg (Ed.), *Maintenance of fluency.* New York: Elsevier.

St. Louis, K., & Lass, N. (1980). A survey of university training in stuttering. *Journal of the National Student Speech, Language and Hearing Association, 11,* 188–197.

St. Louis, K., & Lass, N. (1981). A survey of communicative disorders: Students' attitudes towards stuttering. *Journal of Fluency Disorders, 6,* 49–79.

Schiavetti, N., Sacco, P., Metz, D. & Sitler, R. (1983). Direct magnitude estimation and interval scaling of stuttering severity. *Journal of Speech and Hearing Research, 26,* 566–573.

Schwartz, M. F. (1976). *Stuttering solved.* New York: McGraw-Hill.

Semour, C., Ruggiero, A., and McEneaney, J. (1983). The identification of stuttering: Can you look and tell? *Journal of Fluency Disorders, 8*, 215–220.

Shine, R. E. (1980). Direct management of the beginning stutterer. In W. H. Perkins (Ed.), *Strategies in stuttering therapy*. New York: Theime-Stranton.

Silverman, E., & Zimmer, C. H. (1979). Women who stutter: Personality and speech characteristics. *Journal of Speech and Hearing Research, 22*, 553–564.

Soderberg, G. A. (1962). What is 'average stuttering'? *Journal of Speech and Hearing Disorders, 27*, 85–86.

Tachell, R. H., VanDen Berg, S., & Lehrman, J. W. (1983). Fluency and eye-contact as factors influencing observers' perceptions of stutterers. *Journal of Fluency Disorders, 8*, 221–231.

Van Riper, C. (1973). *The treatment of stuttering*. Englewood Cliffs, NJ: Prentice-Hall.

Webster, R. L. (1974). A behavioral analysis of stuttering: Treatment and therapy. In K. S. Calhoun & K. M. Mitchell (Eds.), *Innovative treatment in psychopathology*. New York: Wiley.

Wendell, R. W., & Cole, J. (1961). Identification of stuttering during relatively fluent speech. *Journal of Speech and Hearing Research, 4*, 281–286.

Wingate, M. E. (1964). A standard definition of stuttering. *Journal of Speech and Hearing Disorders, 29*, 484–489.

Wingate, M. E. (1969). Stuttering as a phonetic transition defect. *Journal of Speech and Hearing Disorders, 34*, 107–108.

Wingate, M. E. (1976). *Stuttering: Theory and Treatment*. New York: Irvington.

Zimmerman, G. (1980). Stuttering: A disorder of movement. *Journal of Speech and Hearing Research, 23*, 122–126.

5

The Psychologically Maladjusted Stutterer*

Michael D. Cox

INTRODUCTION

The psychology of stuttering is less well understood than the physiology of fluency disorder, and the accuracy of scientific measurement is often less precise. The ever-burgeoning literature on the personality and social correlates of stuttering has yet to yield anything approaching consensus on the boundaries between fluency disorder and emotional disorder. A sharp dichotomy exists between those who view stuttering as a result and a symptom of emotional disturbance (Barbara, 1982; Glauber, 1982), and those who view stuttering primarily as a physiologically based disturbance with potential emotional concomitance (Rosenfield, 1984). If stuttering is indeed an overt manifestation of emotional disturbance, then by implication all stutterers are exhibiting signs of significant psychological maladjustment. Fortunately, there is little empirical support for this position. The alternate position more sharply delineates etiology and emotional adaptation by viewing stuttering as a speech mechanism disturbance that has the potential to be emotionally handicapping. Both positions would place the stutterer in a position of abnormal risk for psychological maladjustment.

*This project was supported by the Stuttering Center, The Methodist Hospital and Department of Neurology, Baylor College of Medicine

Stuttering can be conceptualized in two ways: as the result of early emotional trauma that altered the speech mechanism or as a basic physiological defect or vulnerability which is exquisitely reactive to emotional distress. In either instance, future psychological adaptation is dependent upon an individual's status in the family system and society and the individual's ability to cope with the resulting demands, responsibilities, and trauma. Without regard to how the stuttering problem originated, an individual's personal growth and interpersonal development is dependent upon his or her response to this disorder and other significant life events in the framework of their personality organization and interpersonal life circumstance. Whether the etiology of stuttering is anchored in physiological–constitutional factors or emotional disruption, most would agree that this disfluency is an interpersonally handicapping condition and one that represents an unusual burden to an individual's later social adjustment. The degree to which a stutterer is at risk for significant psychological maladjustment is still debated and the interplay of personality and stuttering is still controversial.

DESCRIPTION OF
THE PSYCHOLOGICALLY
MALADJUSTED STUTTERER

A subgroup of the stuttering population clearly demonstrates diagnosable "mental disorder" and social maladjustment. An individual is considered psychologically maladjusted when that individual experiences either painful emotional distress or an impairment in a critical area of behavioral functioning. The most widely accepted conceptualization and criteria for mental disorder or in this case psychological maladjustment, is presented in the third edition of the Diagnostic and Statistical Manual of Mental Disorders (DSM—III) of the American Psychiatric Association (1980). According to this source, a mental disorder exists when an emotionally painful symptom or adaptive impairment is associated with a clinically significant pattern of behavior or psychological syndrome. In other words, an individual is considered psychologically maladjusted when some aspect of his or her behavior is associated with emotional pain or results in impaired adaptive functioning. Adaptive functioning can be viewed as a composite of social-interpersonal relations, occupational functioning, and the use of leisure time. For our purposes, a stutterer is considered maladjusted when the disorder, in conjunction with—or in addition to—other of characteristic behaviors, results in either serious emotional pain or significantly compromised social or occupational functioning. An individual's behavior is always relative to that individual's cultural peers, and an individual can be different from or at odds with society without being considered disordered or maladjusted.

According to this conceptualization, the stutterer is not necessarily damned to significant psychological adjustment problems because of abnormal disfluency. Yet the stuttering population is more vulnerable to maladjustment than are those who do not stutter. This chapter explores the available data and literature pertinent to a subgroup of atypical stutterers considered to be socially and behaviorally maladjusted. Inherent in this schema is the belief that a minority of stutterers demonstrate significant and compromising adjustment pathology. Although this view is certainly not unanimously held, most reviews of the available literature support this conclusion (Bloodstein, 1981; Sermas & Cox, 1982). DSM-III lists stuttering under a subclass disorder referred to as "other disorders with physical manifestation." This subclass includes disorders such as sleep walking, sleep terrors, and functional enuresis. The listing of these syndromes is qualified:

> Inclusion of these categories and classification of mental disorders is justified partly by tradition in that, formally, psychological conflict was sought to play a central role in all of these disorders and it was thought that these conditions were almost always associated with other signs of psychopathology. Recently, however, many have come to question these assumptions, at least with regard to some of these categories. Further, there is evidence that most of the children with these disorders do not have associated mental disorder.

Prevalence of Maladjustment

The prevalance of significant psychological maladjustment in the stuttering population cannot be accurately estimated from our current knowledge. The majority of studies have considered how groups of stutterers compared to groups of nonstutterers on relevant psychological variables and thus were more concerned with the "average" stutterer. To establish prevalence, random selection is necessary, and data collected through clinics, universities, and hospitals are not likely to be representative of the stuttering population as a whole. A portion of the stuttering population at large do not seek assistance for their fluency problem and, therefore, do not surface within the speech service delivery system. Those who present to clinics for help may represent a portion of the stuttering population who perceive themselves as having more adjustment problems, and their stuttering may be more serious. The rate of psychological maladjustment in stutterers who present to speech clinics is likely to be abnormally high. To illustrate, over 50% of those adult stutterers evaluated at the Baylor College of Medicine and The Methodist Hospital Stuttering Center are judged to have significant psychopathology requiring clinical intervention other than speech therapy. The evaluation, consisting of comprehensive psychiatric and psychological examinations, is designed to be especially sensitive to signs of maladjustment, but the population sample tends to be average to high average in socioeconomic status and, therefore, at least occupationally well adjusted.

DESCRIPTIVE STUDIES

The studies of the personality and psychological correlates of the stuttering syndrome are chiefly derived from psychiatric (mainly psychoanalytic) studies, systematic interviews of stutterers and their families, and the application of various psychological personality measures and self-report inventories. Many of the earlier studies did not feature matched comparison groups, but there is a growing volume of literature featuring well-controlled experimental designs. The historical emphasis on personality-oriented research derives from the search for a predictable stuttering personality. The relationship between personality and stuttering marks an area into which "one is drawn intuitively to search for evidence" (Prins, 1972, p. 148) concerning how the two interface. The search for a single, demarcated stuttering personality now appears rather naïve, and the existence of such a personality organization has been challenged over and over again (Bloodstein, 1981; Sermas & Cox, 1982; Sheehan, 1970). Despite the presence of rich and complex literature in the area, the relationship between pertinent personality and psychological variables and the onset, course, treatment, and prognosis of stuttering deserves further clarification.

PSYCHOANALYTIC CONTRIBUTIONS

Although many are quick to discredit the early analytic theorizing, the psychoanalytic study of the stutterer constituted the first logically systematic investigations into the psychology of stuttering, and the resulting data served as a very useful source of testable hypotheses of the personality correlates of stuttering. This method features the intensive study of a smaller number of cases, normally long-term treatment cases, in which the stutterer is seen multiple times per week in individual therapy for several years.

Typically, the psychoanalytic literature regarding stuttering has viewed the disorder as a neurotic symptom underlain by serious psychological conflict. Freud, the founder of the analytic movement, made only two direct statements on stuttering. In 1901 he drew a distinction between slips of the tongue and stuttering by noting that "speech disturbances cannot any longer be described as slips of the tongue because what they effect is not the individual word, but the rhythm and the execution of the whole speech . . . but here too . . . it is a question of an internal conflict which is betrayed to us by the disturbance in speech" (Freud, 1901, pp. 100–101). Thus, Freud thought stuttering to represent an unacceptable instinctual drive. Later he expanded this conceptualization by stating that "stammering could be caused by displacement to speech of conflicts over excremental functions" (Freud, cited in Jones, 1955).

Fenichel (1945) furthered Freud's line of reasoning by pointing out that the stuttering itself was a conversion symptom, that is, a physical displacement and representation of an unconscious conflict. Fenischel considered the basic personality structure of the stutterer to be that of an obsessive–compulsive. Fenischel believed that speech for the stutterer "means, first, the utterance of obscene, especially anal, words and, second, an aggressive act directed against the listener. . . . 'Words can kill,' and stutterers are persons who unconsciously think it necessary to use so dangerous a weapon with care" (Fenichel, 1945, p. 312).

Glauber (1958) departed somewhat from this theorizing by emphasizing the oral elements of stuttering and referring to stuttering as a form of oral arrest. Glauber asserts that the principle trauma in stutterers "is the faulty disallusion of the primary identification with the mother" (p. 337), and he describes the mothers of stutterers as alternately clinging to and rejecting their infants. This early trauma results in both motor and psychological effects and "when a stutterer wants to unconsciously bite or such when he is supposed to speak, a conflict ensues the result of which contains some elements of biting or sucking and also elements of attempts to block or inhibit such expression" (p. 337).

The most extensive psychodynamic theorizing on stuttering is provided by Barbara (1982). In Barbara's opinion, stuttering results from "the anxiety of the stutterer in coping with the world he lives in and in his chaotic attempts to adjust to other people" (p. 4). According to Barbara, the origin of stuttering lies in faulty parenting, in particular, the parents' damaging attitudes and reactions to the manner in which the child speaks. These pathological reactions lead to a "weakened" personality and generate basic anxiety with concomitant feelings of helplessness and anger. The overly distressed parents communicate their anxiety, threats, fears, feelings of overprotectiveness, or feelings of rejection to the child, who in turn focuses too much attention on his or her speech. The act of speaking to another person, then, is converted into a very "self-conscious act" in an atmosphere that generates anger, fear, and threat. As an adult, the stuttering becomes a means of externalizing this same conflict. Barbara believes that "the symptom and the greater part of the ritual of stuttering itself is a major attempt toward an unconscious magic gesture with the purpose of symbolically demonstrating to others how the person who stutters suffers and is victimized" (p. 55). At the same time, Barbara also sees stuttering as an expression of resentment and hostility toward the social environment, which also serves to shield the stutterer from imagined fears of self-anger and aggression.

While Barbara promotes a "neurotic explanation of stuttering," he makes an important contribution to the analytic understanding of stuttering by pointing out the presence of a weakened personality. A theoretical conflict inherent in the neurotic conceptualizations of stuttering exists considering that the onset of stuttering and the faulty parent–child relationship supposedly causing the stuttering occur in the first several years of childhood during which such trauma is thought to result in disorders of self rather than only neurotic disturbances (Kohut, 1971, 1977; Tolpin & Kohut, 1980). Neurosis is the pathogenic outcome of conflicts that occur comparatively later in the child's life, classically during the Oedipal period (ages 4–6), when the child has more firmly established a sense of self. Neurotic symptom formation keys on the presence of an unconscious conflict. A child's libidinal (sexually related) and aggressive drives and impulses create a threatening situation, and this situation generates anxiety. Under the increasing pressure of this anxiety, there is a regression to an earlier stage of development at which the drives have been partially fixated. In turn, the conflictual impulses are rejected and defenses are put into play to suppress and repress them. This suppression and repression are only partially successful, and a psychological compromise becomes manifest in the form of the neurotic symptom (Tolpin & Kohut, 1980). Viewing stuttering as a neurotic symptom neglects the development, the organization, and the condition of the self that underlies and participates in the pathogenic family situation.

In general, the earlier in life and more severe the parent–child trauma, the greater the degree of psychological damage and behavioral maladjustment anticipated as an adult. If indeed the parent–child relationships are seriously disrupted and this disruption occurs in the child's earlier years, than there would be permanent damage to the formation, cohesion, and organization of self, predisposing the child to serious and debilitating forms of psychological maladjustment. So-called narcissistic pathology would be present, and the child would be predisposed to crippling difficulties in the maintenance and regulation of self-esteem, impulse control, identity, trust and intimacy in interpersonal relationships, sexuality, emotional stability, and self–direction. The problem here is that the average stutterer, at least, or stutterers as a population, do not typically show this kind and severity of psychopathology (Bloodstein, 1981; Sermas & Cox, 1982). If the mothers of stutterers chronically cling to and reject their infants as Glauber asserts, then the stutterers would necessarily appear far more maladjusted than they apparently are.

Quite possibly, the analytic writers provide us with an important contribution to the understanding of the atypical stutterer, that is, a stutterer with significant adjustment pathology. Putting aside theory, most stutterers do not appear that seriously maladjusted, but there are a significant number of stutterers who are. The stuttering personality also does not appear to exist (Sermas & Cox, 1982; Sheehan, 1970). Many of the observations and dynamic explanations offered by these theorists may apply to the psychologically maladjusted stutterer. This type of stutterer is unlikely to become fluent when his or her speech is the only focus of treatment and the sole means of treratment concerns the application of better speech controls. The personality defects and painful emotional symptoms limit speech therapy gains that might otherwise be generalized to the individual's social environment. Individuals with significant personality disorder and psychopathology are handicapped in their ability to relate consistently to others in a trusting, intimate, and stable manner. The impostion of a stuttering problem exacerbates this situation. There is great effort and stress involved in learning to speak fluently in interpersonal situations even in the absence of significant psychopathology. The addition of psychological disorder cripples an individual's ability to carryover fluency controls to interpersonal situations which are already disturbing and painful. The psychological maladjustment must also be treated, and a comprehensive psychological understanding of the individual is required.

Descriptive Studies

The major reviews (Bloodstein, 1981; Goodstein, 1958; Sermas & Cox, 1982; Sheehan, 1970) summarily conclude that compared to nonstutterers, stutterers are prone to exhibit lower self-esteem, undue social sensitivity and anxiety, greater fear of occupational and social failure, more social avoidance, and increased diffculty in expressing anger in a direct, adaptive fashion. Obsessional personality trends most often are associated with stuttering, and these concern proneness to tension and worry, emotional overcontrol, reduced self-esteem, over-dependence upon achievement, rigidity, and indecisiveness. These traits are found with more frequency in the stuttering population, but stuttering can be associated with the full range of personality traits and personality organizations. The wealth of descriptive studies now available which compare stutterers to nonstutterers on a variety of personality characteristics seem to converge to two conclusions: There does not appear to be a basic, definable personality associated with stutterers and, on the average, stutterers are only somewhat or mildly more maladjusted than nonstutterers. The reviews of the group comparison studies seemingly downplay the prevalence and degree of psychopathology among stutterers, while the more intense case studies of stutterers tend to overplay at least the etiological role of maladjustment. The fact that stutterers do not differ so drastically from nonstutterers in this regard need not minimize the heightened risk of maladjustment the stutterer faces. The presence of significant psychopathology—whether originating from the social handicap of stuttering or contributing to the onset and maintenance of stuttering—renders the treatment of stuttering extremely difficult. The transfer of within-session fluency gains to the social environment is particularly hampered by psychosocial maladjustment. Stutterers constitute a population at risk for psychological misery and struggle, and to deny this fact is to potentially underserve this population. In most, if not all, cases, stuttering cannot be viewed simply as an encapsulated speech disorder in isolation from personality, as it interacts with the interpersonal-social environment.

Little research has been done comparing subgroups of the stuttering population. Perhaps enough has been done on the interface of personality and stuttering in the traditional sense, but there is certainly a need for research comparing stutterers with one another and comparing stuttering with other fluency disorders,-rather than repetitively comparing stutterers to nonstutterers. To illustrate, no one has yet compared psychologically maladjusted stutterers by any criteria to psychologically well-adjusted stutterers.

The descriptive studies now available may provide direction with regard to how the atypical stutterer demonstrates maladjustment. The known personality correlates of the stuttering syndrome may point the way to psychological pitfalls that the stutterer is vulnerable to and areas of personality formation that are most at risk for developmental arrest. Are there characteristic ways that the stutterer at risk begins to manifest the signs of more intense psychological conflict? Are there certain personality traits, disturbances, or particular constellations of symptoms that are more likely to develop concommitant with the stuttering disorder?

Objective Psychological Testing

The application of standardized psychological tests to assess personality correlates associated with stuttering would intuitively seem a useful and valid approach. Beginning in the 1940s, there was a flurry of research activity in this area, and stutterers were assessed via a multitude of personality tests. Personality tests are usually (and somewhat arbitrarily) subdivided into objective and projective techniques. The objective test restricts the subject's response on standard sets of items to true–false or multiple choice endorsements, while projective tests allow for a more subjective, open-ended, free response format in a comparatively unstructured or ambiguous presentation. Self-report inventories constitute the most common type of objective personality tests. They feature the administration of a standard set of items covering clinically relevant content areas. Each resulting score is regarded as a measure of that content area. By far the most popular and successful of the objective personality tests is the Minnesota Multiphasic Personality Inventory (MMPI). The MMPI was first published by Hathaway and McKinley in 1943 and is still the most widely used test of its kind in clinical as well as research settings. The MMPI is made up of 566 true–false items arranged on 10 clinical scales and three validity scales. Most of the clinical scales were developed from sets of items that statistically differentiated a particular group (e.g., depressed patients) and normal controls. The validity scales measure test-taking attitudes and response sets that may influence and possibly compromise the validity of the clinical scales.

The series of MMPI studies of stutterers has yielded remarkably consistent results. When the MMPI scales are averaged across the stutterers assessed and a group MMPI profile is plotted, the profile tends to fall well within the normal range (Pizzat, 1951; Sermas & Cox, 1982; Thorn, 1949; Walnut, 1954). Stutterers often would have higher clinical scale elevations (in the direction of more psychopathology) than nonstutterers, but these differences did not reach statistical significance and, therefore, the stutterers did not appear to be significantly more maladjusted. The MMPI can be regarded as an objective self-description, and the stutterers do not describe themselves as having more psychological problems than the nonstuttering population. Boland (1953) found that stutterers manifested more symptoms of anxiety as measured on the MMPI, and Walnut (1954) found that stutterers had significantly higher elevations on the depression scale and one other scale (6) that reflects heightened interpersonal sensitivity, distrust, and angry dissatisfaction. In general, stutterers tend to show more anxiety-related psychological distress than nonstutterers when measured in this fashion as a group, but this difference is not clinically significant.

A somewhat different picture emerges when the individual profiles of stutterers are considered. Sermas and Cox (1982) found that 74% of their sample of 19 stutterers had at least one MMPI scale that reached T-score of 70 or greater (a clinically significant elevation). No significant clinical elevation emerged, however, when stutterers were averaged and considered as a group. The unusually high frequency of clinically significant individual scales among the stutterers certainly reflects high rates of psychological distress. The heterogeneity of these elevations, however, suggests that the type of distress and the manner of expression is variable and nonspecific. The abnormal profiles did not hang together in terms of the type or degree of pathology, but personality trait disturbances as well as heightened anxiety and depression were all suggested. The stutterers in this study all presented themselves for speech treatment, and psychosocial distress may have been the major reason for their seeking speech therapy at that time.

Projective Studies

In contrast to the highly structured format and limited response set of the objective measures, projective techniques feature the use of relatively unstructured, ambiguous sets of stimuli allowing an almost limitless variety of individual responses. Free, unbiased responses are encouraged through administration with a minimum of instruction. The central assumption in this type of assessment is that, given an ambiguous stimulus configuration, individuals will perceive, interpret, or organize the configuration according to their distinctive emotional, cognitive, and personality characteristics. Projective techniques are reported to be exclusively sensitive to more covert or unconscious content such as fantasy, needs, impulses, and defensive maneuvers. Projective testing especially lends itself to a more psychoanalytic frame of reference. The emphasis in projective testing is on a global and integrated understanding of the individual.

Projective measures yield a rich and complicated array of individual data. This great harvest of data, however, represents the technique's greatest weakness. Projective techniques are know to be quite subjective and exquisitively reactive to a variety of extraneous examiner and situational influences. Their interpretation is very much dependent upon the skill and sophistication of the clinician, and there can be much variability in interpretation across clinicians. The data can be difficult to quantify, and techniques do not always conform to psychometric standards.

The most popular projective technique is the Rorschach, which continues to be one of the most frequently applied techniques in personality assessment. The Rorschach technique is made up of a standardized set of 10 inkblots, 5 of which are black and white and 5 of which contain color. This technique was first applied to the stuttering population in the 1930s and the 1940s. These studies did not yield anything approaching the consensus found with the MMPI studies. In general, contradictory interpretations arose and opposing conclusions were drawn from much of the same data (Goodstein, 1958; Sheehan, 1958). Many of the studies were accomplished before more detailed and comprehensive scoring systems were available, and the studies focused too narrowly on specific personality traits in conflict areas.

One of the better studies utilizing the Rorschach was that of Santostefano (1960), who evaluated the Rorschach protocols of adult stutterers and nonstutterers for degree of hostility. Although the study lacked blind scoring procedures, it did employ a systematic and validated measure of hostility derived from the content of the subject responses to the blots (Elizur's Rorschach Content Test). Santostefano found significantly more hostility-related content in the protocols of the stutterers. Santostefano interpreted this as a gradual build-up of anger stemming from frustrations of being disfluent. The study, however, has not been replicated.

In the most recent study in which the Rorschach was used with stutterers, Sermas and Cox (1982) found that the Rorschach protocols suggested a variety of conflict areas in their stutterers such as authority, dependency, sexuality, impulse control, and achievement as well as expression of anger. Nevertheless, there was no conflict area or set of conflict areas that characterized their entire sample of stutterers. An as yet unpublished extension of this study found that roughly one-third of the stutterers produced grossly abnormal Rorschach protocols. Once again, these protocols reflected an array of conflict areas, but often the content was most characteristic of an individual suffering from more serious personality disorders. Remarkably, these findings did not correlate with the results from the objective tests of personality. In other words, many of the individual stutterers who produced grossly abnormal Rorschachs also produced MMPI profiles technically within normal limits. These stutterers did not view themselves as having significant psychological problems even though clinical interviews found evidence of significant interpersonal problems. In addition, the stutterers producing the pathological Rorschachs did not evidence the degree of disturbance characteristic of the most maladapted personality organizations, even though they certainly appeared to have more social difficulty than they viewed themselves as having. The abnormalities found on their Rorschachs, then, may suggest the degree of underlying injury, frustration, and conflict in a subset of stutterers who are not particularly comfortable with self-disclosure and tend to rationalize and deny their level of accumulated distress.

The Rorschach is also a perceptual device. An alternative explanation to the Rorschach abnormalities found in a subset of stuttering population may concern differences in stutterers' perceptual organization. Several investigators (Cox, 1982; Smith & Daley, 1980) found evidence of larger and more frequent Wechsler Adult Intelligence Scale (WAIS) Verbal-Performance IQ differences, most often in the direction of lesser performance than verbal IQs. The WAIS Performance IQ has a strong perceptual organization factor, and the fact that this score is lowered with some stutterers may suggest divergent perceptual organization (not necessarily deficient or impaired). Therefore, the Rorschach abnormalities could be related to perceptual differences rather than personality factors.

The second most popular projective technique, the Thematic Apperception Test (TAT), also has been used to assess the personality characteristics of stutterers. The subject is required to make up a story from a series of cards depicting a variety of scenes. This technique has produced rather equivocal results with adult stutterers, but a similar technique used with children (Children's Apperception Test) has elicited indications of heightened suppression and anxiety in child stutterers (Wyatt, 1958, 1969).

To summarize the psychological test findings, stutterers as a group seem to suffer from mildly elevated anxiety, sensitivity, and insecurity in social situations together with somewhat lowered self-image and difficulties in expressing anger in an adaptive fashion. Serious psychological maladjustment does not appear to be a typical circumstance for the stutterer, and, on the average, stutterers do not appear at risk for major psychopathology. Those stutterers who are maladjusted do not appear to be abnormally prone to the psychotic syndromes (e.g., schizophreniform illness) or major affective disorders. Rather, these stutterers experience anxiety-related symptomatology, mild to occasionally moderate levels of depression, and impaired social functioning. The maladjusted stutterer also is especially vulnerable to significant self-image defects and, at the extreme, serious disorders of self and personality trait disturbances.

Stuttering Children and Their Families of Origin

Child stutterers also do not exhibit substantial psychological maladjustment, although there is ample conflicting evidence here as well. Child stutterers tend to be regarded by their parents and others as more anxious, socially insecure, and emotionally reactive than their nonstuttering peers. Mild academic problems such as underachievement also seem to be more prevalent in childhood stutterers as a group (Bloodstein, 1981). Child stutterers do not appear to be at any greater risk for seriously debilitating psychopathology than their fluent peers.

The parents of stutterers have been studied extensively in the past and they do not appear to be a particularly disturbed group (Goodstein, 1966). In his review of the literature on the parents of stutterers, Bloodstein (1981) concludes that the parents are somewhat more inclined to be anxious, perfectionistic, domineering and to set high expectations for their offspring. In a large study of MMPI profiles of parents ($N = 447$) of stuttering children, Goodstein and Dalstrom (1956) determined that the MMPI profiles of the stutterers parents did not differ significantly from those of control parents or the test norms. Goodstein and Dalstrom conclude:

> There was no evidence that the etiology of stuttering is rooted in the gross psychological pathology of the stutterers' parents but rather the results are to be interpreted as supporting the notion that such attitudes and adjustments of the parents as may be involved in the etiology of stuttering are probably limited and specific to the speech situation. (p. 370)

Goodstein (1956) confirmed these findings in a follow-up study. In a later review article, Goodstein (1958) concluded that the existing differences between parents of stuttering children and parents of fluent children were not suggestive of gross maladjustment of parents but centered around "subtle attitudes of perfectionism and criticalness" (p. 366), and these attitudes specifically related to the speech area.

Although abnormally high rates of gross psychopathology do not seem to be the case, those studies finding evidence of maladjustment in childhood stutterers and their families might provide a view of the atypical, maladjusted stutterer and the developmental and family systems origins of that maladjustment. Most theories of psychopathology place the origins of that pathology in defective parenting and family system disorder, constitutional and genetic contributions notwithstanding. Accordingly, psychologically maladjusted stutterers differ from their more adequately adjusted, nonfluent peers in terms of their fortune in early childhood.

Certainly, maladjustment can originate from unusual and intense stress occurring in adulthood in cases where the early childhood experience and family background appear adequate and stable. Yet when substantial and sustained maladjustment is precipitated in adulthood, the person often has been rendered more vulnerable to this maladjustment because of the traumas and inadequacies of support in his or her childhood. To illustrate using an actual case, a 39-year-old stutterer is plunged into a self-image crisis with clinically significant levels of anxiety, depression, and social withdrawal following a divorce. His wife's dissatisfaction with the marital relationship came as a surprise and a shock to the stutterer, and he found himself unable to resolve the loss of his wife and his accustomed home environment. The stutterer became increasingly listless at work, self-disparaging, and socially isolated. His catastrophic reaction to the divorce and its aftermath is better understood in the context of a history of earlier loss. The stutterer lost his mother when she suffered severe trauma in a fall when he was 11 and his father from an apparent suicide when he was 16. These losses, particularly the loss of his father, were not adequately mourned, and his divorce occurred in the same month as his father's death. His most recent loss reactivated the unresolved injury and distress associated with the loss of his parents, and his reaction was understandably intensified to a pathological degree. His speech concomitantly worsened, and psychotherapy plus subsequent speech therapy were initiated.

The onset of stuttering often has been associated with traumatic events occurring within the family. Sermas and Cox (1982) reported that approximately 60% of their stutterers recalled stressful circumstances related to the onset of their speech difficulties. For example, one of their stutterers became nonfluent at 7 years of age, when his father's alcohol abuse became apparent. The stutterer recalled having difficulty sleeping at night because his father was banging on the piano and swearing loudly. Another of their patients began stuttering at 3 years of age, while his mother was hospitalized. This stutterer first had difficulty with his speech when he spilled the contents of a pot of coffee, seriously burning himself. Also at the age of 3, another patient pulled his younger brother off the bed causing the infant to scream out in fright. The terrified 3-year-old ran to the kitchen to inform his mother. The child found that he was unable to speak fluently, and he continued to stutter thereafter.

Another patient was 5 years of age when his father lost his job and began drinking heavily. The loss of the job necessitated the child's mother working outside the home, and frequent quarrels ensued between the parents when she returned from work. The stuttering first occurred during that period, and the stutterer's father continues to blame himself for his son's speech problem.

Such background data is anecdotal, and such information cannot be used to link the cause of stuttering to acute family trauma or misfortune. The presence of family distress, however, can indicate significant family system dysfunction, which can significantly alter the child's adjustment. In this respect, Ierodiakonou (1970) studied 65 stuttering children (3–15) without the benefit of a comparison group. He found that 75% of his sample experienced psychologically traumatic events associated with the onset of stuttering, most often eliciting reactions of terror in the child. The intensity and frequency of these traumatic events led the author to deem stuttering as "exceptional among those neurotic or psychosomatic" (p. 173) disorders, as the stuttering is precipitated by trauma rather than developed gradually over time. The precipitating event was often related to parental attitudes that aggravated the stuttering condition. The author also noted that most of his stuttering sample already has shown evidence of psychological maladjustment, and he described the prestuttering personality as "very insecure and sensitive to criticism" (p. 173). He also found eating problems to be a frequent and concomitant symptom.

Despert (1946), in his case study of 50 child stutterers and their parents, found that many of his subjects listed traumatic events as causative factors in their stuttering. The author felt that these events could be viewed as precipitating events, even though he found a wide variation in speech pathology and age of speech onset. Similarly, Glasner (1949) reported a high incidence of disturbing, precipitating events in the family environments of his 70 childhood stutterers. Glasner noted that "the disruptive influence of grandparents, aunts, or other relatives" (p. 137) was frequently found, and that removal from the source of this distress often led to the resolution of the stuttering. Glasner did not find evidence of basic psychological maladjustment in his sample of stutterers, however. Bryne, Willerman, and Ashmore (1974) believe that their language-impaired children are more likely to have experienced potentially traumatic environmental influences. Robbins (1964) also found that parents of stutterers often linked early trauma to the development of their children's stuttering.

The presence of alcoholism certainly represents serious and disabling trauma to a family system as a whole and the children in particular.

Sermas and Cox (1982) were surprised to find that 42% of their small sample (19) had a close relative that clearly abused alcohol. This finding has been sustained in a larger but yet unreported sample, and this finding deserves independent replication. Most of the patients' fathers were reported to be abusing alcohol when the stuttering began. Alcohol abuse clearly can be associated with family stress, and alcoholism and affective (depression-related) mental disorder have been linked genetically.

The reported precipitating traumas of stuttering vary in kind and intensity. Not all stutterers began their stuttering in traumatic circumstances, and not all the children experiencing emotional traumas of this sort go on to become significantly maladjusted as adults. If the precipitating trauma does not occur in isolation and the family system is dysfunctional, then the individual developing within this situation would have a higher vulnerability to later maladjustment.

At least one researcher attributes stuttering to "a specific ego dysfunction" that is "socio-genetically transmitted . . . by the nuclear family" (Wertheim, 1973, p. 155). Based upon the study of 16 stutterers' families and 16 control families, Wertheim concludes that this ego dysfunction in conjunction with certain self-interpersonal perceptions and language patterns provide a sufficient condition for the development of stuttering. In these stutterer's families, language is used not only as a means of communication but as a "tool of interpersonal power assertion" (p. 171). Wertheim further theorizes that a dyad emerges in families of stutterers, most frequently the father–son dyad. This fosters "power deprivation" (p. 172) in the stuttering child, which is instrumental in the maintenance of stuttering behavior.

Such writing sounds rather strident in condemning parents and their attitudes as the cause of stuttering. Research addressing the etiological role of parenting in the development of stuttering is neither in particular agreement, nor is the research itself of sufficient quality and comprehensiveness to draw such conclusion. Moreover, considering the evidence for genetic contributions and physiological differences, it is certainly inaccurate and even cruel to site parents as the main cause of a child's stuttering. Mental attitudes influence the course of stuttering (Quarrington, 1974), and defective parenting may predispose to psychological maladjustment in general. For example, a child who is abused physically, sexually, or emotionally within the family will be at risk for later defective self-esteem and self-organization, depression, interpersonal mistrust, interpersonal instability, and deficient impulse control. A child who is genetically vulnerable to stuttering because of a strong family history of stuttering and who is also abused within the family will be predisposed to the same type of pathology. The abused child, whether speech fluent or disfluent, also will be more at risk for mistreating their own children because of the role socialization within their families of origin and their lack of adequate parent role models. Parents who were themselves abused normally do not want to be defective and damaging in their parenting, but such parents often lack the necessary psychological well-being, training, and resources to be effective parents.

A child's position within a family may influence the parent–child relationship as well. Rotter (1939) and Sermas and Cox (1982) found a trend toward greater separateness in age between the stutterer and other siblings. Rotter conducted the largest study of this kind by analyzing the family positon of 522 male and female stutterers. Rotter found significantly more only children and fewer middle children in his stutterers than among the general population. Rotter also reported that the number of years between the stutterers and their nearest sibling was significantly greater than the mean number of years between the stutterers' fluent siblings. Rotter reasoned that, if a child is separated by several years from the nearest sibling the parents have more time to focus on that child. If indeed the parents of stutterers tend to be more overprotective, anxious, perfectionistic, and demanding (Despert, 1946; Glasner, 1949; Moncur, 1952), then such a child may be more at risk to be adversely influenced by such attitudes. Such attitudes could influence the child toward a poor self-concept, dependency, underassertiveness, and inadequate social self-confidence. Stuttering, of course, would be seen as but one form of maladjustment emanating from such circumstance.

The self-concept of stuttering children would appear to be particularly vulnerable. Wallen (1973), studying stuttering and nonstuttering adolescents, found that the stutterers had lower self-concepts than their fluent counterparts. Wallen also found that the ideal self-image of the stutterers was lower than that of the non-stutterers. Moncur (1955) found evidence of anxiety and insecurity, which could certainly predispose a stutterer to a deficient self-concept. Moncur studied stuttering children ages 5–8 years using parental reports of symptomatology. Compared to a matched and fluent sample, the stuttering children displayed significantly more symptoms of distress. Moncur states that "young stutterers characteristically appear to be very nervous, or enuretic, have nightmares and night tears, display aggressive behavior, or claim to be 'fussy' eaters and need to be disciplined often" (p. 96). Since these findings were based upon parental report, it may be that parental attitudes and characteristics are biasing factors in this type of reporting.

The innate behavioral tendencies of the child also will determine to some extent how the environment will react to that child. Thomas and

Chess (1977) view temperament as a characteristic behavioral style for the child, beginning in the first few weeks of life. In this way, temperament encompasses an organismic rather than an environmental contribution to individual psychosocial development, emphasizing how a child reacts, not why. Such reactivity is reflected in the areas of activity level, rhythmicity, adaptability, mood, reaction, intensity, responsiveness, distractability, and attention. "Easy" children are generally positive (exhibit likable behavior) in these areas, while "difficult" children are negative, and "slow-to-warm-up" children show a mixture of positive and negative behaviors. Parental and other environmental interactions with an easy child tend to be positive, while difficult children are frustrating and environmental interactions are often negative, putting these children at greater risk for unfavorable development. Several of the preceeding authors (Glasner, 1949; Ierodiakonou, 1970; Moncur, 1955) have noted behavioral problems in children that could suggest greater proportions of more difficult or slow-to-warm-up children among their sample of stutterters. This type of child interacting with difficult parents may create a highly conflictual environment, predisposing the child to later maladjustment.

To summarize, significant psychological maladjustment of the stutterer later in life would seem to be associated with earlier family system conflict and pathological parent–child interactions. The presence of sustained trauma in a family, as against more acute and isolated incidents, is more likely to be associated with later psychological maladjustment rather than simply serving as a precipitating event. There also appears to be a subgroup of stutterers who demonstrate behavioral symptoms other than speech-related defects who are more at risk for adult psychological problems. The child'd developing sense of self is particularly sensitive to early injury, and adult stutterers are likely to show primary difficulties in this area. Family system dysfunction and developmental disorder may not necessarily predispose to stuttering but certainly predisposes to maladjustment whether an individual stutters or not.

IDENTIFICATION OF MALADJUSTMENT

Identification of individuals experiencing psychological maladjustment is normally accomplished through interviewing, behavioral observations, and psychological testing, if the last is available. Obviously, the skills and experience necessary to diagnosis psychopathology accurately normally lie beyond the training of a speech–language pathologist. Yet the speech–language pathologist must be sensitive to the presence of significant maladjustment even though proper evaluation, diagnosis, and treatment planning may have to be carried out by a psychologist, psychiatrist, or appropriately trained social worker. The questions become when to make an informed referral and when concomitant psychotherapy intervention is necessary. An individual who stutters most often presents multidimensional problems, and the treatment of this individual is often multidisciplinary in nature. The multidisciplinary approach to stuttering should be more the rule than the exception.

Psychologically maladjusted stutterers in most cases will identify themselves through their own self-reports and behavior. The speech–language pathologist must listen, ask the proper questions, and become acquainted with the whole person. Adult stutterers will often seek speech therapy during times of transition and when they are experiencing heightened interpersonal and/or occupational stress. A very important question to ask these individuals is "Why are you seeking therapy at this particular time?" Many will answer that their fluency has declined or that they have a greater need for improved speech at this time. The issue then becomes the identification of life stress related to speech decline and major social or occupational change indicating the presence of a transitional period.

A stuttering child will often be referred either by his or her parent or by a teacher when there is elevated distress in the family system. From a family systems perspective, the onset of stuttering in a child who is physiologically vulnerable or a decrease in fluency in a child who already stutters may be viewed as symptomatic of increased distress in the family constellation, much as the child who acts out rebelliously at school is reflecting family-based conflict. As we have seen before, stuttering is often precipitated by trauma occurring within a family. The question remains: Why is his or her speech changing now? and What has happened in the family that may be associated with this change?

An older stutterer may respond to an upsurge in psychological stress in his or her life through increased focus on the struggle for fluency and seek speech therapy. The stutterer may place the cart before the horse in noting that his or her fluency has deteriorated and attribute most if not all of the increased psychological stress to the speech disorder. A corresponding wish is expressed that if only the disfluency would resolve, than other life-related problems would relent. In such cases, it is necessary to identify the other related or unrelated problems in a person's life and to treat both the speech and the person's method of coping with life's responsibilities and stressors.

The most direct way to identify a stutterer who is experiencing significant adjustment problems is through interviewing that person or the parents and siblings in the case of the young child. The interview must include the stutterer's current life circumstance and adjustment plus a personal history. An i ndividual should be asked whether there are any current sources of stress, conflict, or significant dissatisfaction in his or her life. Direct questions concerning the adequacy of an individual's marital, social, and occupational adjustment should be asked. Does the person have enough close friends? Have there been any recent personal losses? Have there been any recent occupational changes or reversals? Is the person satisfied with his or her dating relationships or marriage? Has there been any decline in social contact or activity?

The personal history should survey familial relationships, psychiatric history in the family or the individual, scholastic achievement and adjustment, establishment of independent functioning apart from the family, social-interpersonal adjustment, occupational adjustment, the emotional climate in the family of origin, drug usage, and medical history. In the case of children, parents should be queried about the presence of temper tantrums, nightmares, phobias, enuresis, developmental delays, feeding problems, adequacy of relationship with parents, relations with siblings, and the general emotional climate in the family and in the marriage. Once again, the child can serve as the symptom-bearer for a family or a marriage that is in distress. In school-age children, downturns in level of socialization, school performance, and/or increased rebelliousness are usually telltale indications of psychological distress.

The presence of debilitating anxiety and depressed mood can be readily identified through interview. A person can be queried with regard to the amount of worry, tension, nervousness, and anxiety in his or her life and in which areas the anxiety is the greatest. Has the stutterer ever experienced anxiety so acute and intense that he or she became panicked and feared loss of control? There is a strong relationship between anxiety and speech disfluency, and, as noted earlier, stuttering is an affect-sensitive disorder.

Depressed mood is often characterized by reports of feeling sad, down, low, "blue," despondent, hopeless, gloomy, and so on. Clincially depressed individuals may manifest a host of characteristic symptoms that may include sleep disturbance, difficulty falling asleep, restless sleep pattern or early awakening, changes in appetite with weight loss, decreased ability to experience pleasure, decline in energy, decreased sexual interest, decreased interest in work and usual activities, lessened self-confidence, lowered self-esteem, feelings of helplessness, increased irritability, decreased ability to concentrate, lowered short-term recall and forgetfulness, pessimism, thoughts of death, and suicidal ideation. If there is any reason to suspect suicidal ideation, the stutterer should be asked directly and frankly about self-destructive thoughts, the presence of any plans to commit suicide, any history of attempts, and any history of suicide within the family or among significant others.

The point is not to subject each stutterer who comes through the door to an intrusive clinical interview. Enough personal information should be gathered to screen for obvious maladjustment and to understand the individual one is dealing with. Adequacy of social and occupational adjustment has important ramifications for treatment planning, response to treatment, and whether or not other professionals need to be involved in the treatment. Sufficient information must be gathered in order to allow an informed referral in the case of serious maladjustment.

The stutterer with underlying psychopathology may manifest difficulties through a poor response to treatment. The stutterer who is not well motivated and is resistant to treatment often is having difficulties adjusting in other areas of life as well. The stutterer who stumbles as the transfer stage of therapy begins may well have deficient coping skills. The stutterer who is unable to organize sufficiently to practice on a consistent basis may show a similar degree of organizational problems as he or she confronts other life responsibilities.

Psychopathology can manifest itself in terms of a rapid and a tense transference reaction within speech therapy. Speech–language pathologists and the stutterer normally form a close, working relationship as the therapy progresses. Transference refers to patterns of anticipations and expectations developed in past significant relationships that form the basis for current, meaningful relationships. Transference involves the displacement or "transfer" of fantasies, thoughts, attitudes and feelings onto the person in the present that were originally a part of relationships with significant others in the past, most often parents. Preconceived attitudes are imparted to the therapist. Counter transference refers to the therapist's displacement of preconceived attitudes derived from childhood experience onto the patient. Transference is a ubiquitous phenomenon that can be either positive or negative. Transference occurs in all person-to-person relationships and more intensely in relationships that are enduring and have emotional significance. Evidence of transference generally unfolds gradually and, in more dynamic therapy where the patient is seen several times a week over an extended period of time, a transference neurosis is fostered. This type of transference reaction involves the recapitulation of the same maladaptive behavior, traits and coping mechanisms that originated in the parent–child relationship. In speech therapy, rapid and intense appearance of unwanted and unwarranted feelings of anger, love, and sexuality may signal the presence of significant psychological disorder. When this type of reaction occurs early in the speech therapy, a more primitive personality organization is usually present and psychotherapy is usually called for.

TREATMENT CONSIDERATIONS

In most cases, the psychologically maladjusted stutterer will need concomitant therapeutic intervention other than speech therapy and, in some cases, the other therapeutic intervention may have to preceed involvement in speech therapy. The resolution of the psychological maladjustment and increased disfluency is unlikely to occur through speech therapy alone. Intervention focused on the speech disfluency will not remediate the interpersonal maladjustment that in turn works against the transfer of fluency controls to the social environment. Gains made in the therapy session are less likely to generalize to the outside world, and relapse is more likely to occur. Transfer is the most critical phase of speech therapy, and speech controls learned in the supportive therapy relationship must ultimately generalize to society where the demands, anxieties, and responsibilities are so much greater. An individual who has difficulty coping effectively with life's stresses and demands and who struggles in relationships even apart from speaking difficulties may have neither the ability nor the motivation necessary to transfer speech therapy gains. The presence of such maladjustment will certainly impede transfer over time and heighten the risk for premature termination of speech therapy.

Psychotherapy directed at the "whole person" is less likely to resolve the stuttering in the absence of intervention directed at speaking differently. Whether behaviorally, analytically, or family systems–based, psychotherapeutic intervention promotes personal growth and enhanced coping ability in relation to life's demands. To the extent that dysfluency is associated with impaired interpersonal functioning and social adaptation, psychotherapy aimed at personal growth also will be speech beneficial. Stuttering is not simply a neurotic symptom, and even therapies directed at symptom relief are not likely to produce fluency. Psychotherapy can lay the foundation, alay psychological obstacles, and generally pave the way for the applicatins of speech therapy gains.

A psychologically maladjusted stutterer most often requires a joint and coordinated effort among disciplines. Speech therapy and psychotherapy normally can be concomitant, but stutterers who are more severely disordered or in acute distress may require initial involvement in psychotherapy prior to speech training. In cases of serious depression, frequent panic attacks, or emotional instability, psychotherapeutic intervention is required up front.

The combined therapeutic effort normally required for the comprehensive treatment of the psychologically maladjusted stutterer necessitates cooperation and mutual understanding among therapists. Therapeutic roles must be clearly delineated and the boundaries and limits of the therapeutic interventions clearly defined with the patient (if old enough) and between the therapists. Devisive splitting can occur where there is ambiguity and a lack of coopertive exchange among the therapists providing services to the individual patient. Certain patients, particularly those with a personality disorder, can attempt consciously or otherwise to create division between therapists by blurring the boundaries between one therapeutic relationship and another (e.g., talking critically about the psychotherapist to the speech pathologist). Therapists must not collude with the patient in these types of splitting interactions, and the patient should be encouraged to deal with their feelings toward their therapist most directly (e.g., the patient should be encouraged to express his or her dissatisfaction directly to the psychotherapist rather than "triangling-in" the speech–language pathologist). Mutual respect and understanding across disciplines is essential for the combination approach to be effective.

The following sections detail therapeutic interventions that are particularly helpful in the case of the psychologically maladjusted stutterer. The majority of these interventions require specialized training and experience beyond that normally provided a speech pathologist. When working comprehensively with this type of stutterer, it is important that these additional interventions be available in the community. Networking is urged wherein consultative liasons with other professionals are developed and nurtured.

SUPPORTIVE THERAPY

The atypical maladjusted stutterer will likely require increased emotional support, whether this support is provided within the speech therapy relationship or in supportive psychotherapy with a mental health professional. Supportive interventions are designed to control the symptoms of psychological maladjustment while fostering socially adaptive behaviors. Expressing concern and reassurance for an individual and promoting socially rewarding behavior and problem solving that changes environmental circumstances to reduce stress are supportive interventions certainly not restricted to mental health professionals. Supportive interventions have much in common with the counseling an individual receives from a trusted clergyman, mentors, family members, close friends, and significant confidants, whom Schofield (1964) has called the invisible therapists. Supportive therapy is often sufficient to resolve stress and improve adjustment when an individual's personality organization is basically sound and the problems encountered are the result of overwhelming, environmentally-based stress. When the problems are more deeply rooted and pervasive, more intensive and uncovering approaches may be necessary to promote the necessary personal growth. Supportive therapy works best with individuals who are reasonably stable, have been involved in at least one sustained and intimate relationship, voice fairly specific complaints, and remain motivated to change. There are other patients for whom supportive therapy is the only reasonable alternative because more intense insight-oriented therapy is either unavailable or too intense and overwhelming for the patient. These patients have a long history of, at best, marginal adjustment and poor interpersonal relationships.

Supportive therapy is directed toward the "here and now," and the goal is to suppress anxiety and alleviate stress. The therapist avoids exploration of the potential dynamic underpinnings of conflicts and symptoms. The purpose is not *personality* change so much as enhanced utilization of personal and environmental resources to effect *positive* change. Insight-oriented or uncovering psychotherapy can be thought of as more anxiety provoking, intensive, and in-depth. The insight-oriented approaches refer to psychoanalysis, psychoanalytically oriented individual psychotherapy and short-term dynamic psychotherapy. The goal of insight-oriented psychotherapy is intrapsychic change and the reorganization of personality through the recognition and expression of unconscious conflict (Sermas & Scnekjian, 1982). In this type of therapy, the client is seen multiple times per week, and the client must have the capacity for insight and the ability to tolerate the anxiety evoked. Often the therapist challenges the patient's behavior in order to help the patient explore more openly the disguised conflicts in childhood injuries that perpetuate stress. As Sermas and Scnekjian note, the message in supportive psychotherapy is "Don't be afraid, because you can do it," while the strategy in uncovering psychotherapy is "Let's see what really makes you fearful."

The most frequently applied supportive techniques are ventilation, reassurance, guidance, and environmental manipulation (Sermas & Scnekjian, 1982). The patient is encouraged to open up within a trusting relationship and voice his or her complaints, distress, and painful feelings. The act of expressing personal doubts and fears allows patients to confront distortions and to develop a more constructive attitude toward themselves and their problems. The fact that the therapist does not reject the patient, despite the revelation of personal doubts and shortcomings, promotes a better acceptance of self. This assurance should be offered on both a verbal and nonverbal level, that is, a therapist's behavior must be consistent and aligned with the therapist's verbal statements. Missed appointments, unreturned phone calls, frequent interruptions of the session, and casualness on the part of the therapist deplete therapeutic effectiveness up to the point of premature termination. Reassurance must be genuine and pertinent and never ingratiating and false. Reassurance can be inappropriately used to suppress a patient's emotional ventilation that the therapist finds too anxiety provoking. The most common applications of reassurance include reassuring the patient that his or her symptoms and problems are not unique, that the patient can make significant improvement, that the symptoms are painful but not dangerous (e.g., anxiety panic reaction), and that the patient is not totally losing control or falling apart emotionally. Guidance is provided in supportive psychotherapy by means of fact giving, interpretation, and instruction. More realistic and adaptive courses of action are suggested by a therapist who is an authority and possesses expertise. Guidance can counter impulsivity and poor judgment, which only exacerbate a person's problems. A thoughtful discussion and examination of the patient's circumstances can lead to positive environmental manipulation on the part of the patient to provide more support and positive input. The presence of a trusted and respected therapist allows the patient to "bounce off" the therapist ideas, potential decisions, and feelings.

Stress Management And Anti-Anxiety Measures

The most recent National Institute of Mental Health (NIMH) (1984) studies found that anxiety (followed by substance abuse and then depression) is the most common mental health problem in the United States. Stuterers are expecially vulnerable to excessive anxiety, and when their anxiety levels increase, their fluency and social adjustment typically decline accordingly.

One of the most effective approaches to anxiety control is the development of stress management skills. In stress management training, the individual works toward acquiring specific techniques for decreasing the negative and painful impact of stress-producing life events. Stress management often can be accomplished through a short-term, small group program, but some stutterers will require a more intensive, individual format. Stress management normally includes relaxation training, self-assessment and self-monitoring techniques, visual imagery training, cognitive restructuring, assertiveness, and time management training. An individual learns to define stress and the psychological and physical impact of that stress. The individual also learns how he or she reacts to stress and how to identify the sources of stress in his or her environment. Through training in relaxation, positive mental imagery, assertiveness, time management, and the elimination of negative self-statements and negative anticipations, the person learns alternative and more adaptive responses to stressful situations.

Biofeedback training can often complement and enhance stress management training. During biofeedback training, individuals obtain feedback about selected physiological responses, and this feedback, in turn, is helpful in learning to control these responses and lessen reactivity to daily stress. Biofeedback in and of itself, however, typically does not provide a sufficiently comprehensive approach to anxiety reduction.

Particularly intense or pervasive anxiety can be treated with the addition of short-term courses of minor tranquilizers, referred to as anxiolytics and benzodiazepines. Medication for anxiety is best prescribed by a psychiatrist, and the medication should be used in conjunction with stress management training or other therapeutic interventions. The anxiolytics certainly reduce anxiety temporarily, but drugs do nothing to instruct the patient on how to deal more effectively with life stress. Moreover, the anxiolytics carry side effects including sedation, decreased concentration, poor coordination, tolerance and physical addiction with high doses, and withdrawal syndromes (usually mild).

GROUP THERAPY

Supportive group therapy is particularly valuable and applicable to maladjusted stutterers. Group therapy can also be intensive and insight oriented, but the focus generally is on more supportive measures with this population. The focus of supportive group psychotherapy is the same as that found in individual therapy, that is, symptomatic remission and promotion of more effective social functioning. The group approach is particulary valuable because it allows stutterers to work constructively with one another on the basis of a shared experience. Unfortunately, resistance to self-disclosure and behavioral change are common among stutterers. To a greater degree than in individual therapy, stutterers in a group format can learn that their symptoms and situations are not unique and that their fears, self-doubts, and anxieties are shared by others. Stutterers can uniquely support each other in a manner that is not available in other therapeutic approaches. A group can generate more powerful motivation for the sustained effort required for fluency and related social change.

Group therapy inherently is interpersonal in focus, and a stutterer's interpersonal behavior is observed as it emerges in the development of the group. In this way, the group functions as an interpersonal laboratory in which relationships are formed. The stutterer forms relationships with his or her peers as well as the cotherapists in their roles as authority figures. The group provides, therefore, an excellent base to work on the transfer of speech controls to the real world environment and enhance social adjustment in general. Yalom (1975) proposes a set of curative factors that are relatively common to all group approaches. These curative factors fall into 11 categories: installation of hope, universality, imparting of informaton, altruism, corrective recapitulation of primary family group, development of socializing techniques, imitative behavior, interpersonal learning, group cohesiveness, catharsis, and existential factors.

Cotherapists, rather than a single therapist, and the most effective means of leading a group. A particularly helpful combination is that of a speech pathologist who has had group experience and a psychologist, psychiatrist, or social worker. This combination imparts concerned expertise with the joint areas of speech fluency and interpersonal-social adaptation. Optimal group size in this case parallels that of other groups and is normally around six to eight participants, excluding therapists.

FAMILY THERAPY

Intervention at the family systems level (family therapy and marital therapy) should be available when working with the maladjusted child stutterer. A child cannot be considered in isolation from the family. The onset of stuttering can follow from stress in the family and exacerbations of disfluency can be caused by family-based conflict. The family can be viewed as the patient in this type of therapy. The maladjusted family system is seen as the cause of a psychological problem, and the identified patient is considered the symptom bearer for the family. The exacerbation of disfluency in a child will be considered a product of the total family problem. A young stutterer who is showing more struggle with speech, school adaptation, and social functioning may be responding to family pressures by providing a cover for his parents' marital conflict. The pathogenic process in the family may be defined and explored during the therapy sessions in which family members interact characteristically. The goal of this type of therapy is to assist family members in identifying and modifying the roles, structures, and communications that form the genesis of the identified patient's symptoms. Marital and couples therapy are most often viewed as another aspect of the family systems approach, since the couple is a basic dyad in the family unit. Family therapy requires a therapist with special skill and experience in this type of approach, and intervention should not be attempted without the necessary training.

SUMMARY

The majority of evidence favors the view that stuttering is a physiologically based disorder that is affect sensitive and exquisitely reactive to anxiety. Stuttering can be considered a psychosomatic disorder, since the onset and course of stuttering is influenced by psychological factors, both internal and external. Existence of the "stuttering personality" or dominant personality organization associated with stuttering has not received empirical support. There is little evidence to suggest that stuttering is simply a psychological symptom that is underlain by more basic emotional conflict.

A subgroup of the stuttering population clearly demonstrates diagnosable mental disorder and social maladjustment. The psychologically maladjusted stutterer, however, does not appear abnormally at risk for psychotic syndromes, major affective disorders, or the most severe personality disorders. Stutterers considered as a population are more prone to excessive anxiety, compromised self-image, social avoidance, undue social sensitivity, decreased ability for emotional self-disclosure, and difficulties in expressing negative affect than nonstutterers. The psychologically maladjusted stutterer is likely to have significantly more problems in these areas than the average stutterer, and the maladjusted stutterer is particularly vulnerable to debilitating self-esteem pathology.

A multidisciplinary approach is recommended, and the psychologically maladjusted stutterer usually needs concomitant psychotherapeutic intervention other than speech therapy. The resolution of the psychological maladjustment is unlikely to occur through speech therapy alone, and the resolution of the speech disfluency is unlikely to occur through psychotherapy alone. Stress management training and group psychotherapy are particularly valuable and applicable to this population.

In the case of the maladjusted child stutterer, psychotherapeutic intervention at the family systems level should be considered. Family system function and the adequacy of relationships with parents and siblings should be assessed. The onset of stuttering is often associated with stress within the family, and a child's behavioral maladjustment as well as decreased fluency may be considered a reflection of family system conflict.

REFERENCES

American Psychiatric Association. (1980). *Diagnostic and statistical manual of mental disorders* (3rd ed.). Washington, D.C.

Barbara, D. A. (1982). *The psychodynamics of stuttering.* Springfield, IL: Thomas. (1981).

Bloodstein, O. N. (1981). *Handbook on stuttering.* Chacago: National Easter Seal Society.

Boland, J. L. (1953). A comparison of stutterers and nonstutterers on several measures of anxiety. *Speech Monographs, 20,* 144.

Bryne, B. M., Willerman, L., Ashmore, L. L. (1974). Severe and moderate language impairment: Evidence for distinct etiologies. *Behavioral Genetics, 4,* 331–345.

Cox, M. D. (1982). The stutterer and stuttering: Neuropsychological correlates. *Journal of Fluency Disorders, 7,* 129–140.

Despert, J. L. (1946). Psychosomatic study of 50 stuttering children. *American Journal of Orthopsychiatry, 16,* 100–113.

Fenichel, O. (1945). *The psychoanalytic theory of neurosis.* New York: Norton.

Freud, S. (1901). *Psychopathology of everyday life.* New York: MacMillan.

Glasner, P. J. (1949). Personality characteristics and emotional problems in stutterers under the age of five. *Journal of Speech and Hearing Disorders, 14,* 135–138.

Glauber, I. P. (1958). Freud's contributions on stuttering: Their relationship to some current insights. *Journal of American Psychoanalytic Association, 6,* 326–347.

Glauber, I. P. (1982). *Stuttering: A psychoanalytic understanding.* New York: Human Sciences Press.

Goodstein, L. D. (1956). MMPI profiles of stutterers' parents: A follow-up study. *Journal of Speech and Hearing Disorders, 21,* 430–435.

Goodstein, L. D. (1958). Functional speech disorders and personality: A survey of the research. *Journal of Speech and Hearing Research, 1,* 359–376.

Goodstein, L. D., & Dahlstrom, W. G. (1956). MMPI differences between parents of stuttering and nonstuttering children. *Journal of Consulting Psychology, 20,* 365–370.

Hathaway, S. R., & McKinley, J. C. (1943). *The Minnesota Multiphasic Personality Inventory.* New York: Psychology Corporation.

Ierodiakonou, C. S. (1970). Psychological problems and precipitating factors in the stuttering of children. *Acta Paedopsychiatr (Basel), 37,* 166–174.

Jones, E. (1955). *The life and work of Sigmund Freud.* New York: Basic Books.

Kohut, H. (1971). *The analysis of the self.* New York: International Universities Press.

Kohut, H. (1977). *The restoration of the self.* New York: International Universities Press.

Moncur, J. P. (1952). Parental domination in stuttering. *Journal of Speech and Hearing Disorders, 17*, 155–165.

Moncur, J. P. (1955). Symptoms of maladjustment differentiating young stutterers and nonstutterers. *Child Development, 26*, 91–96.

Pizzat, F. J. (1951). A personality study of college stutterers. *Speech Monographs, 18*, 240–241.

Prins, D. (1972). Personality, stuttering severity, and age. *Journal of Speech and Hearing Research, 15*, 148–154.

Quarington, D. (1974). The parents of stuttering children. *Canadian Psychiatric Association Journal, 19*, 103–110.

Robbins, S. D. (1964). 1,000 stutterers: A personal report of clinical experience and research with recommendations for therapy. *Journal of Speech and Hearing Disorders, 29*, 178–186.

Rosenfield, D. B. (1984). Stuttering. *CRC Critical Reviews in Clinical Neurobiology. 1*, 117–139.

Rotter, J. B. (1939). Stuttering in relation to position in the family. *Journal of Speech Disorders, 4*, 143–147.

Santostefano, S. (1960). Anxiety and hostility in stuttering. *Journal of Speech and Hearing Disorders, 19*, 220–227.

Schofield, W. (1964). *Psychotherapy: The purchase of friendship.* Englewood Cliffs, NJ: Prentice-Hall.

Sermas, C. E. & Cox, M. D. (1982). The stutterer and stuttering: Personality correlates. *Journal of Fluency Disorders, 7*, 141–158.

Sermas, C. E. & Senekjian, M. A. (1982). *Supportive treatment: Basics of therapeutic care.* in H. S. Moffic and G. L. Adams (eds.), *A clinician's manual on mental health care: A multidisciplinary approach.* Menlo Park, CA: Addison-Wesley.

Sheehan, J. G. (1958). Projective studies of stuttering. *Journal of Speech and Hearing Disorders, 23*, 18–25.

Sheehan, J. G. (1970). *Personality approaches* in J. G. Sheehan (ed.), *Stuttering: Research and therapy.* New York: Harper and Row.

Smith, A., & Daly, D. A. (1980). *Neuropsychological assessment: Implications for treatment of aphasic and stuttering clients.* Mini-seminar presented at the American Speech-Language-Hearing Association Convention, Detroit.

Thomas, A. and Chess, S. (1977). *Temperament and development.* New York: Brunner and Mazel.

Thorn, K. F. (1949). *A study of the personality of stutterers as measured by the MMPI.* Unpublished doctoral dissertation, University of Minnesota.

Tolpin, M., & Kohut, H. (1980). The disorders of the self: The psychopathology of the first years of life. In S. I. Greenspan & G. H. Pollock (Eds.), *The Course of Life: Psychoanalytic contributions toward understanding personality development: Vol. 1. Infancy and early childhood.* Washington: National Institute of Mental Health.

Walnut, F. (1954). A personality inventory item analysis of individuals who stutter and individuals who have other handicaps. *Journal of Speech and Hearing Disorders, 19*, 220–227.

Wyatt, G. L. (1958). A developmental crisis theory of stuttering. *Language & Speech, 1*, 250–264.

Wyatt, G. L. (1969). *Language, learning, and communication disorders in children.* New York: Free Press.

Wallen, V. (1973). A Q-technique celluose of the self-concepts of adolescent stutterers and nonstutterers. *Child Development, 26*, 91–96.

Yalom, I. (1975). *The theory and practice of group psychotherapy.* New York: Basic Books.

6

The Mentally Retarded Stutterer

Eugene B. Cooper

Stuttering among the mentally retarded, as in all atypical populations, offers us opportunities to increase our understanding of the various factors that affect fluency. With such understanding, we are able to serve all disfluent individuals more effectively. Unfortunately, as the review of literature in this chapter reveals, very little research in the past decade focused on the fluency of the mentally retarded. If this lack of research effort continues, opportunities for increased understanding of stuttering will be lost. Perhaps publications such as this one, drawing attention to the dearth of research in this area, will stimulate renewed interest in stuttering in the mentally retarded individual.

While little research on the nature of stuttering in the mentally retarded has been reported in the recent past, significant strides continue to be made in the development of therapeutic procedures and materials applicable to the mentally retarded stutterer. A number of commercially available programs have been designed for clinicians working with stutterers. Techniques and materials useful with mentally retarded individuals of varying degrees of retardation in varying age groups are included in some of those programs. Thus, while lagging research efforts may curtail opportunities to increase our understanding of stuttering, our ability to provide effective and efficient treatment to many mentally retarded stutterers has increased significantly.

The purpose of this chapter is to review what research has been re-

123

ported concerning stuttering in mentally retarded populations, to discuss the implications of the results of that research, and, finally, to describe diagnostic and therapeutic techniques, procedures, and materials found to be useful with mentally retarded stutterers. The chapter begins with a brief review of classifications used in defining mentally retarded populations. It continues with a review of studies indicating the prevalence of stuttering in mentally retarded populations and a discussion of the nature of the stuttering observed in such populations. Issues such as differentiating between the mentally retarded stutterer and clutterer and determining when stuttering therapy for the retarded is warranted are discussed. The chapter continues with a description of diagnostic and therapy procedures and materials that have been found to be useful with the retarded stutterer. It concludes with a discussion of service delivery systems applicable to the mentally retarded stutterer.

THE MENTALLY RETARDED

Definition

According to the American Association on Mental Deficiency (AAMD), mental retardation "refers to significantly subaverage general intellectual functioning resulting in or associated with concurrent impairments in adaptive behavior and manifested during the developmental period" (Grossman, 1983, p. 11). The AAMD definition of significantly subaverage is related to an IQ of 70 or below on standardized measures of intelligence. The developmental period is defined as the period of time between conception and the eighteenth birthday.

Classification Systems

Table 6.1 presents the AAMD's most recent classification system for determining levels of retardation. Obviously the term *mental retardation* is used to encompass a heterogeneous population ranging from the totally dependent to the nearly independent. According to the AAMD (Grossman, 1983) the identifiable mentally retarded population can be divided into two groups. The first group, constituting approximately 25% of the total population, demonstrates some central nervous system pathology, typically has IQs in the moderate range or below, has assorted handicaps or stigmation and can be diagnosed from birth or early childhood. The second group, typically identified during the school years, appears neurologically intact, has no readily detectable physical

Table 6.1
Level of Retardation Indicated by IQ Range Obtained on Measure
of General Intellectual Functioning[a]

Term	IQ range for level
Mild mental retardation	50–55 to approx. 70
Moderate mental retardation	35–40 to 50–55
Severe mental retardation	20–25 to 35–40
Profound mental retardation	Below 20 or 25

[a]Adapted from H. J. Grossman (Ed.), *Classification in mental retardation.*
Washington, DC: American Association on Mental Deficiency, 1983.

signs related to retardation, functions in the mildly retarded range of intelligence, and is heavily concentrated in the lowest socioeconomic segments of society.

Another classification system used primarily for educational purposes and dependent typically on IQ scores uses the terms EMR (educable mentally retarded), TMR (trainable mentally retarded) and S/PR (severely/profoundly retarded). Individuals classified as EMR are considered to be mildly retarded (50–75 IQ), and those classified as TMR are considered to be moderately retarded (35–50 IQ). The S/PR category includes those individuals with IQs of 35 or below. According to Blackhurst and Berdine (1981), this system is currently the most useful one for special education programming.

Other classification systems frequently used are those based on etiology and those based on clinical type, which attempt to separate symptoms of the retardation from its causes (Mandell & Fiscus, 1981). Regardless of what type of classification system is used in grouping the mentally retarded, there is universal agreement that the mentally retarded should be classified only when such classification leads to the development of appropriate programs to meet the needs of the individual involved.

Prevalence and Incidence

Estimates as to the prevalence of mental retardation vary markedly. The AAMD (Grossman, 1983) reports figures ranging from 2 to 3%. A 3% prevalence figure indicates that over 6 million individuals in the United States could be classified as mentally retarded. However, Grossman notes that many individuals with IQs below 70 who are regarded as retarded during school age lose the diagnosis in adulthood. While estimates of the prevalence of mental retardation varies markedly, there appears to be a consensus that the incidence of mental retardation in the United States is at about 125,000 births per year.

PREVALENCE OF STUTTERING
IN THE MENTALLY RETARDED

As might be predicated with such a heterogeneous and ill-defined group as the mentally retarded, estimates of the prevalence of stuttering in that population very markedly. Bloodstein (1981) summarized the results of prevalence studies dating from 1912 through 1978 (See Table 6.2). No additional prevalence studies concerned with identifying stutterers in mentally retarded populations have appeared in the literature in the United States since that time. Inspection of Table 6.2 reveals that the occurrence of stuttering was found to vary from as little as 0.8% (Sheehan, Martyn, & Kilburn, 1968) to as high as 20.3% (Schlanger, 1953a, 1953b) in institutions for the mentally retarded. If the currently popular 0.7% stuttering prevalence figure in the general population is accepted, the prevalence of stuttering was found to be higher than in the general population in *all* of the mentally retarded populations studied. Bloodstein (1981) concluded: "Stuttering, apparently of all degrees of severity and complexity, would seem to occur more frequently in this population than in any other single identifiable group of people" (p. 162).

Review of the studies noted in Table 6.2 reveals that the prevalence of stuttering increases as the severity of retardation increases within retarded populations possessing expressive speech competencies. This relationship can be observed easily in the Brady and Hall (1976) and the Boberg, Ewart, Mason, Lindsay, and Wynn (1978) studies in which the prevalence of stuttering in the TMR groups is about twice as great as in the EMR groups (see Table 6.2).

The prevalence of stuttering in mentally retarded individuals with Down's syndrome deserves special attention. With the exception of the Martyn, Sheehan, and Slutz (1969) study in which only one stutterer was observed among 42 Down's syndrome subjects, investigators have found the prevalence of stuttering in that population to be unusually high. Gottsleben (1955) found a prevalence rate of 33%, while Schlanger and Gottsleben (1957) observed a 45% prevalence rate of stuttering in individuals with the Down's syndrome. Lubman (1955) found a 21% prevalence rate in a population of 48 children with the Down's syndrome. Van Riper (1982, p. 41) cites Edson (1964) as reporting a 45% prevalence figure and Schubert (1966) as reporting a 15% prevalence

Table 6.2
Prevalence of Stuttering among Persons with Mental Deficiency[a]

	N^b	Population	Percent-age of stutterers
Ballard (1912)	944	Special school for mentally defective children	2.4
Louttit & Halls (1936)	620	Ungraded classes for subnormals	3.22
Wohl (1951)	145	Special schools for mentally and physically handicapped	5.5
Karlin & Strazzulla (1952)	50	Outpatient hospital clinic for retarded children	2.0
Schlanger (1953)	74	Institution for mentally retarded	20.3
Schlanger & Gottsleben (1957)	516	Institution for mentally retarded	17.0
Stark (1963)[c]		Educationally subnormal children	10.0
Schaeffer & Shearer (1968)	4,307	Institution for mentally retarded	7.6
Sheehan, Martyn, & Kilburn (1968)	216	Institution for mentally retarded	0.8
Martyn, Sheehan & Slutz (1969)	346	Institution for mentally retarded	1.0
Chapman & Cooper (1973)	1,467	Institution for mentally retarded	3.02
Brady & Hall (1976)	3,057	Educable mentally retarded	1.6
Brady & Hall (1976)	457	Trainable mentally retarded in schools	3.08
Boberg et al. (1978)	840	Classes for educable mentally retarded	1.43
Bobert et al. (1978)	439	Classes for trainable mentally retarded	2.51

[a]Reproduced from Bloodstein, O. *A Handbook on Stuttering*. Chicago: National Easter Seal Society, 1981.
[b]Where data were obtained in institutions. N refers to the total number in the survey population who had speech.
[c]Cited by Andrews and Harris (1964, p. 7).

figure for the occurrence of stuttering in individuals with Down's syndrome. Van Riper (1982, p. 40) also notes that Keane (1970) found a 10% prevalence figure in his unpublished study. Subsequently, Keane (1972) reviewed the studies to that time that dealt with the incidence of speech–language problems in the mentally retarded. On the basis of all of these reports, it appears safe to conclude that stuttering is found among individuals with Down's syndrome at an unusually high rate (Zisk & Bialer 1967). Several of these investigators raise the issue as to whether the disfluencies observed in the Down's syndrome population should be labelled *stuttering* or *cluttering*. That issue is discussed the next section of this chapter.

THE NATURE OF STUTTERING IN THE MENTALLY RETARDED

This section begins with a review of studies concerned with the nature of stuttering observed in general populations of mentally retarded individuals. Following that is a review of studies concerned specifically with the nature of stuttering observed in individuals with Down's syndrome. The issue of whether the fluency problems observed in Down's syndrome populations (and in at least a portion of the general mentally retarded population) is stuttering or cluttering is then discussed. The section concludes with a summary of what currently appears to be the most defendable observations on the nature of stuttering in the mentally retarded.

Stuttering in General Populations of the Mentally Retarded

Schlanger and Gottsleben (1957) studied the speech of the total population of 516 residents at a state institution for the mentally retarded. These subjects included 377 males and 139 females with a mean chronological age of 28.9 years and a mean mental age of 7.8 years. They applied the terms *clonic, tonic,* and *secondary reactions* to those subjects judged to be stutterers. Eighty-nine of those subjects (17%) stuttered. Schlanger and Gottsleben observed repetitions (clonic blocks) in 92% and prolongations (tonic blocks) in 57% of the stutterers. Secondary reactions were observed in 26% of their stuttering subjects.

Lerman, Powers, and Rigrodsky (1965) studied the fluency and reactive patterns of 14 mentally retarded institutionalized stutterers. Their ages ranged from 9.5 to 17.6 years and their mental ages ranged from 4.2 to 8.9 years. Lerman et al. concluded that the children they observed revealed patterns generally void of reactive symptoms and demonstrated stuttering patterns "resembling the early stages of stuttering development" (1965, p. 27).

Chapman and Cooper (1973) observed stuttering behavior in 36 of 1467 residents of a state institution for mentally retarded persons. Of these 36, 18 completed testing procedures for measuring adaptation, consistency, and expectancy. The 18 subjects were selected on the basis both of their ability to complete the testing procedures and of the demonstration of stuttering behavior on at least 10% of the stimulus pictures. The age of the 18 subjects ranged from 12 to 78 years, with a mean age of 35.6 years. The subjects' IQ's ranged from 20 to 62, with a mean IQ of 40.3. The length of institutionalization for the subjects ranged from 8 months to 48 years, with a mean of 18.8 years.

Chapman and Cooper (1973) found evidence to suggest the existence of the adaptation, consistency, and expectancy phenomena in the stuttering of the mentally retarded. They found the frequency of stuttering in the first presentation of 25 stimulus pictures decreased approximately 43% by the fifth presentation of the pictures. Individual consistency percentages based on the formula suggested by Tate and Cullinan (1962) ranged from 0 to 48% with a mean of 29.29%. The group consistency rate was found to be 36%, which is less than half of the consistency rates frequently cited in the literature (Bloodstein, 1981). Although only five of their subjects indicated expectancy of stuttering, stuttering occurred on 100% of the words on which it was expected. Stuttering occurred on 34% of the words on which it was not expected by those same five subjects, with individual percentages ranging from 16 to 50. Chapman and Cooper suggested the subjects' relative inability to indicate expectancy might have been related to testing procedures rather than to any lack of stuttering expectancy in the subjects. Subjects were required to make responses (tapping to indicate expectancy) that required cognitive processing. The investigators noted that an assessment of expectancy through physiological measurements such as heart rate, skin resistance, or palmar sweat would have more accurately indicated the presence or absence of the expectancy phenomena. Chapman and Cooper concluded that their data suggest "the stuttering behavior of the mentally retarded stutterer is subject to the same laws as that behavior of the nonretarded stutterer with respect to the adaptation, consistency, and expectancy phenomena" (1973, p. 157).

Bonfanti and Culatta (1977) compared the fluency patterns of 32 institutionalized, mentally retarded adult stutterers to the patterns of 10 severely retarded adults not diagnosed as stutterers and to the descriptions of narmally intelligent disfluent children and normally intelligent disfluent adults. Bonfanti and Culatta found that both their stuttering and nonstuttering retarded groups exhibited disfluency rates that would place them in the "severe" stuttering category (12–25% of the words spoken). They found the retarded adults to evidence a predominance of syllable, word, and phrase repetitions in contrast to only rare occurrences of revisions, broken words, or blocks. Secondary characteristics were observed but judged to be minimal. They contrasted the frequency of occurrence of the various disfluency types (interjections, part-word repetitions, revisions, etc.) they observed in their retarded groups with the frequency rates observed by Yairi and Clifton (1972) in the disfluencies of preschool children. Bonfanti and Culatta found no significant relationship between the disfluency frequency types found in their retarded adults and frequency types observed in preschool children. They did note, however, that there was a stronger relationship between disfluency frequency types between stuttering retarded adults and non-stuttering retarded adults than there was between those two groups and the disfluency frequency types observed in preschoolers.

Bonfanti and Culatta (1977) observed that only one-third of their subjects were able to define stuttering verbally, although two-thirds of the subjects accurately identified other residents who stuttered. They also reported their subjects "generally seemed unconcerned with their disfluencies. Specifically there was little or no evidence of postponement, avoidance of words or sounds, or visual signs of frustration or anxiety following disfluency episodes" (p. 127). They concluded that retarded adult stutters are aware of their lack of fluency but are not concerned about it.

Stuttering in Down's Syndrome Populations

Cabanas (1954) observed the fluency of 50 Down's syndrome subjects ages 5–15 over a 2-year period. He characterized their disfluent speech pattern as cluttering, since he observed them to have insufficient vocabularies, hurried speech patterns, and a lack of ideo-motor equilibrium. He observed no self-consciousness or self-observation in the children's behavior and found no indications that the children anticipated difficulty with their fluency or made any effort to avoid disfluencies.

Preus (1973) studied 67 Down's syndrome individuals above the age of 7 in two Norwegian institutions for the mentally retarded. Of the 47 individuals on whom Preus reports data, 35 were between the ages of 10 and 27 and the IQs ranged between 20 and 60, with a mean IQ of 38. Ten judges who knew the subjects listened to recordings of the subjects responding to various test stimuli. The listeners were asked to indicate the types of disfluencies they heard on the tapes and to judge, on the basis of their knowledge of each subject, the presence or absence of secondary symptoms, stuttering or cluttering. Eighty-one percent of the subjects exhibited whole-word repetitions, 85% part-word repetitions, and 64% prolongations. Thirty percent of the subjects exhibited secondary symptoms that Preus defined as body movements, avoidance, and postponement. Preus interpreted these findings as indicating those clients were consciously experiencing the problem of stuttering.

Otto and Yairi (1975) obtained spontaneous speech samples of 19 institutionalized nonstuttering individuals with Down's syndrome and of 19 normally intelligent individuals. The institutionalized subjects (9 males and 10 females) ranged in age from 14 to 31 years, with a mean age of 21 years, 4 months. The group's mean IQ was 36. Members of the normal group ranged in age from 15 to 32 years with a mean age of 22.4 years. The tape-recorded speech samples were analyzed to determine the frequency of occurrence of disfluency types and the proportion of each category in the total number of disfluencies in each subject's speech. Otto and Yairi observed no significant differences between the nonstuttering Down's syndrome group and the normal group with respect to total disfluencies. However, the occurrences of part-word repetitions, disrhythmic phonations, and tension were noted to be significantly greater in the Down's syndrome group, while the proportion of interjections to the total number of disfluencies was found to be significantly higher in the normal populations. Otto and Yairi concluded that "Down's syndrome is often associated with disfluent speech patterns where 'stuttering-like' elements are rather pronounced while elements of 'normal' disfluency, though still present in a considerable amount, are relatively de-emphasized. In other words, even nonstuttering mongoloids speak in a manner which is favorable to the development of stuttering" (1975, p. 30).

Farmer and Brayton (1979) studied 13 Down's syndrome individuals whose mean chronological age was 30 years, 8 months (SD 9 yr, 4 mo) and mean mental age was 7 years, 7 months (SD 1 yr, 2 mo). The investigators observed the subjects' articulation intelligibility ratings and disfluencies, as well as the vowel duration of the subjects' vocalizations of 12 three-word phrases and sentences designed for obtaining vowel duration measures. On the basis of the number of disfluencies observed, the subjects were divided into a fluent group of seven subjects and a disfluent group of six subjects. No significant differences in articulation scores were found between the fluent and disfluent group. However, significant differences were found between the two groups with respect to vowel duration, frequency of disfluencies, and intelligibility. The disfluent Down's syndrome subjects displayed a pattern of "fairly good articulatory scores on single-word responses, poor intelligibility in conversational speech, frequent disfluencies and shorter vowel duration" (1979, p. 288).

Stuttering and Cluttering

Throughout the literature concerning stuttering in the mentally retarded, investigators have raised the question as to whether the disfluencies observed in the mentally retarded are symptoms of stuttering or cluttering. The question is particularly prevalent in the discussions of disfluencies in individuals with Down's syndrome, apparently because of the assumption of underlying physiological differences in that population. Daly describes the problem of cluttering in detail in Chapter 7, this volume. However, a brief definition of cluttering appears appropriate here to assist the reader in understanding the issue of stuttering versus cluttering in the mentally retarded. According to Weiss (1964), cluttering is a central language disorder characterized by short attention span, impaired articulation, a rapid speech rate with frequent breaks in the following of speech, and a lack of awareness on the part of the speaker to those speech abnormalities.

Early writers suggesting the disfluencies noted in the mentally retarded are symptomatic of cluttering rather than stuttering, based their thinking on their observations that few if any disfluent retarded speakers indicate an awareness of their disfluencies (an awareness that the writers assumed to be a primary characteristic of stuttering). Cabanas (1954), for example, found no evidence of anticipations, substitutions, or other avoidance devices in 50 disfluent Down's syndrome individuals. On the basis of such observations, he argued that the disfluencies resembled cluttering more than stuttering.

However, as the review of literature above indicates, subsequent evaluations of disfluent mentally retarded speakers suggest that avoidance behaviors and other indications of awareness were observed, at least to some extent, in all the studies in which this function was assessed. For example, Schlanger and Gottsleben (1957) reported "secondary reactions" in 26% of their subjects; Chapman and Cooper (1973) observed the expectancy phenomena in their retarded disfluent subjects; and Bonfanti and Culatta (1977) reported that their subjects were aware of their disfluency but unconcerned about it. Preus (1973) observed behavior in 30% of his Down's syndrome population, which he interpreted as indicating an awareness to and a reaction to the disfluencies being experienced.

Preus (1973), in the study noted previously, attempted to differentiate stutterers from clutterers in his population of Down's syndrome subjects. On the basis of the judgment of a panel of 10 judges who knew the subjects involved, Preus concluded that between 34 and 47% of his 47 subjects would be labeled stutterers, and between 11 and 40% could be labeled clutterers. It is difficult to determine the exact criteria on which the judges relied in making their judgment. It appears, however, that suttering was defined as the presence of repetitions and prolongations, accompanied by behaviors suggesting reactions to the disfluencies. Cluttering was defined primarily as rapid speech, misarticulations, and intelligibility.

After reviewing these studies, it is apparent that elements purported to characterize both cluttering and stuttering appear in significant proportions in mentally retarded disfluent populations, including those with the Down's syndrome. Van Riper (1982), in musing as to whether the mentally retarded disfluent individual should be labeled a stutterer or a clutterer, noted:

> If we accept Weiss' (1964) position that all stuttering begins as cluttering (which we do not) then the problem of differential diagnosis presents no problem-many of these children clutter. They show the accompanying language deficits, the misarticulations, the reversals, the lack of fear or awareness that characterizes cluttering. . . . If stuttering represents the final common path of a group of related disorders, a syndrome, one which arises in cluttering and language disability, then this is the type of stuttering that the mentally retarded show.

Summary Observations

Most, if not all, of the significant published studies of stuttering in the mentally retarded are noted above. Little reflection is required to conclude that our pool of knowledge is meager and much is left to be discovered. From these studies, however, an indication begins to emerge of the scope of the problem of stuttering in the mentally retarded, as do glimmers of the nature of stuttering in the population. Such information provides us with tentative guidelines for intervention.

It is appropriate to summarize what we know about the prevalence of stuttering as well as the nature of stuttering in the mentally retarded. The prevalence of stuttering is higher in mentally retarded populations than it is in any other known population. The prevalence of stuttering increases as the severity of retardation increases, when nonspeaking mentally retarded populations are excluded from consideration. A significant number of the disfluent mentally retarded demonstrate behaviors indicating awareness of the speech abnormality if not concern with the disorder. The types of disfluencies exhibited by the disfluent mentally retarded stutterer are similar to those observed in populations of stutterers of normal intelligence. A significant number of mentally retarded disfluent individuals (particularly those with Down's syndrome) also exhibit behaviors such as abnormally rapid speech and articulatory disorders characteristic of the syndrome labeled cluttering. Phenomena such as adaptation, expectancy, and consistency, which are observed in populations of stutterers with normal intelligence, are also observed in a significant number of the mentally retarded stutterers. Thus, it appears that much of the stuttering behavior observed in the mentally retarded is similar to that observed in stutterers of normal intelligence. In addition, as would be expected in a population with central neurological deficits, the stuttering behavior is frequently accompanied by language, phonological, articulatory, rate, and fluency problems characteristic of the clutterer.

DIAGNOSTIC CONSIDERATIONS

This section describes the viability of providing speech, language, and hearing services to the mentally retarded and then discusses the goals of diagnostic and assessment activities with these individuals. The section concludes with descriptions of assessment materials applicable to disfluent mentally retarded children and adults.

Viability of Services for the Mentally Retarded

In November 1981, the American Speech–Language–Hearing Associations's Legislative Council adopted as an official statement of the Association a position paper entitled "Serving the Communicatively Handicapped Mentally Retarded Individual" (ASHA, 1982). The statement notes that prior to 1960 the prevailing attitude was that mentally retarded people did not benefit from services provided by communicative disorders specialists. It reviews the history of the development of programs for the mentally retarded in the 1960s, with the New Frontier and Great Society programs of Presidents Kennedy and Johnson, respectively, as well as the growing community conscience of the American people. The position statement continues with a description of how federal laws passed in the 1970s (PL 93-380, Education Amendment of 1974; PL 94-142, The Education for All Handicapped Children Act of 1975; and Section 504 of PL 93-112, Rehabilitation Act of 1973) mandated far-reaching changes in services to the mentally retarded population. These laws required services to all handicapped persons in the least re-

strictive environment. As a result of these developments, mentally retarded persons of all ages are now being served by communicative
disorders specialists in the many environments (e.g., residential facilities, public schools, sheltered workshops) where the mentally retarded
are found. The ASHA position statement reaffirms the profession's
commitment to serve these individuals, and describes the role of the
speech–language pathologist and the competencies needed to meet the
communicative needs of the mentally retarded. Thus, as never before,
communicative disorders specialists are being provided the opportunity
to serve the mentally retarded.

According to ASHA's (1982) position paper, the role of the communicative disorders specialists providing services to the mentally retarded
includes:

1. Assessing, describing, and documenting the communicative behaviors and
   needs of each client and interpreting and integrating the communicative needs
   with educational and vocational programming.
2. Evaluating various modes of communication with reference to the individual's abilities, disabilities, and communicative environment, in order to develop the most effective means of communication possible, vocal and
   otherwise.
3. Developing speech and vocal communication to the fullest extent possible,
   while placing preeminence on the development of language rather than just
   speech.
4. Developing intervention procedures and evaluating their effectiveness in
   producing systems of communication which meet the communication demands of the environment, interface with other programming, and are appropriate to educational, vocational, and social settings.
5. Incorporating within assessment and intervention program procedures "significant others" in the life of the mentally retarded individual including: direct caregivers, family members, employers and other professional team
   members.
6. Where necessary, training persons to interact with the mentally retarded person who uses an augmentative system of communication. (p. 550)

The mandate is clear. Professionals practicing speech–language
pathology and audiology in the discipline of human communication sciences and disorders are committed to providing quality comprehensive
services to assist the mentally retarded in maximizing their communication skills.

Diagnostic Goals

One of the more difficult questions confronting speech–language clinicians working with mentally retarded stutterers is "When is therapy
for the individual's fluency problem indicated?" For many of the dis-

fluent mentally retarded, stuttering appears to be a minor annoyance in comparison to their other communication problems. In addition, as noted above in the review of studies concerning the nature of stuttering in the mentally retarded, many of the disfluent individuals are unconcerned about their stuttering. Such realities, while upon first reflection discouraging to the speech clinician wishing to facilitiate the development of fluency skills, provide guidelines for determining the efficacy of stuttering therapy for the mentally retarded.

Clinicians determine whether a fluency-facilitating intervention program should be undertaken by answering the following questions:

1. What is the nature of the disfluencies observed?
   a. What type of disfluencies are observed (e.g., part-word repetitions, whole-word repetitions, phrase repetitions, hesitations, or prolongations)?
   b. What is the frequency and the consistency of the disfluencies?
   c. Is the expectancy and adaptation phenomena observed?
2. What is the relative significance of the disfluencies to the total communicative competency of the individual?
3. What is the individual's perception of the significance of the disfluencies?
4. To what extent would fluency-enhancing strategies, if adopted by the client, positively effect other aspects of the individual's speech intelligibility (rate, stress, articulation, voice)?
5. What are the constraints placed upon an intervention program with respect to such variables as time, place, frequency of contact, length of sessions, individual versus group sessions, and continuity of services?
6. What is the prognosis for a sustainable enhanced fluency?
7. To what extent will an increased fluency enhance the individual's ability to communicate and thereby improve the individual's quality of life?

While some of these questions are relatively easy to answer, others require clinical judgments that, given our present state of knowledge, must be based on guesswork at best. Until our discipline provides us with such answers, which appears doubtful in the forseeable future, clinicians will continue to struggle with such questions. Fortunately for the mentally retarded, the number of support systems for maximizing the efficiency and effectiveness of intervention programs on their behalf has increased significantly since the early 1960s. More frequently today than in the past, the work of communicative disorders specialists with the mentally retarded is being reinforced by the placement of the mentally retarded in life situations that foster increased communication skills. Thus, it is more relevant today than ever before that speech-language pathologists do all they can to assist the mentally retarded in realizing their full potential with respect to their ability to communicate.

Significance of Cognitive and Affective Responses to Assessment

Embedded in the diagnostic goals discussed above is an acknowledgement of the significance of the mentally retarded stutterer's attitudes and feelings to the development of intervention strategies. Daly (1977) and Guitar and Bass (1978) presented data to support the frequently reported clinical observations (Cooper, 1984) of the significant relationship between attitude changes and long-term stuttering therapy outcome. Such a relationship appears to exist in the mentally retarded stuttering population as well. In fact, the relationship between attitudes and maintenance of fluency may be more easily observed in mentally retarded populations. Clinical observations suggest mentally retarded stutterers, unless they have the potential to or are capable of expressing feelings and attitudes about their communicative behavior, typically are unable to sustain the fluency elicited in the clinical situation. Consequently, attending to the client's attitudes and feelings is a critically important aspect of any fluency assessment undertaken to determine the efficacy of initiating an intervention program.

The Frequency Fallacy and Assessment

Bloodstein (1981), after a comprehensive review of procedures used to assess the severity of stuttering, concludes that listener judgment appears to be the single most valid measure. He also notes the apparently limitless number of variables that appear to effect changes in an individual's disfluency rate at any given point in time. Such observations led Cooper and Cooper (1985) to conclude that stuttering frequency may be the single *least* reliable and valid measure of stuttering severity. They suggest that for too long, too many clinicians have judged stuttering severity and client progress in therapy on the basis of a "frequency fallacy" that assumes frequency to be the best measure of stuttering severity. In overzealous attempts to arrive at numbers on which to base clinical decisions, clinicians and researchers too frequently overlook the unreliability and clinical meaninglessness of stuttering frequency counts obtained in clinical situations. The misuse of stuttering frequency measures can be observed easily in therapy programs that use such counts as stuttered words per minute to determine when a client is ready to move from one activity to another and to determine when clients can be enrolled or dismissed from therapy. Obviously, the frequency of disfluencies is a significant factor in the measurement of stuttering behavior. However, for the reasons noted above, disfluency frequency counts should not be the keystone of stuttering assessment procedures.

Assessment Instruments

The need to focus on broader issues than the frequency of stuttering when evaluating the disfluent individual is apparent. The diagnostic and assessment instruments described below reflect the attempt to assess fluency in the context of the individual's total communication pattern. Because, as noted previously, so many mentally retarded individuals exhibit more than one type of communicative disorder, it is assumed a comprehensive speech, language, and hearing evaluation will be completed on every disfluent mentally retarded client. The instruments described here are aimed specifically at the fluency aspects of the client's speech and language behavior.

Cooper and Cooper (1985), in their *Cooper Personalized Fluency Control Therapy—Revised* (PFCT-R) program materials, present fluency assessment digest and treatment plan protocols for both children and adults. Both of these protocols may be used with nonreading, lower-functioning children and adults. These instruments, as the authors note, are based on the assumption that the measurement of stuttering severity must include not only its behavioral components in all their complexity, but the client's cognitive and affective responses as well. One comprehensive and multidimensional approach to the diagnosis and assessment of stuttering can be described by reviewing the contents of the children's and the adolescent and adult fluency assessment digests developed by Cooper and Cooper (1985)

Children's Fluency Assessment Digest

The "Cooper Personalized Fluency Control Therapy—Revised (PFCT-R) Assessment Digest and Treatment Plan—Children's Version" (Cooper & Cooper, 1985) is a 16-page booklet that includes, for the convenience of the clinician, both assessment and treatment plans (as does the adolescent and adult version). Included in the 12-page assessment digest portion of the booklet are the knowledge assessment instruments:

Chronicity Prediction Checklist
Parent Assessment
Teacher Assessment
Frequency Assessment
  Recitation
  Responding
  Repeating
  Reading
  Picture Identification
  Elicited Spontaneous Speech
Duration of Stuttering Moments
Concomitant Behaviors
Attitudinal Indicators of Significance of Stuttering
Situation Avoidance Reactions
Child's Perceptions of Severity
Clinician's Perceptions of Severity

The first page of the booklet, in addition to providing client identification data, is for summarizing the data obtained in each assessment activity. Following is a description of each of the assessment instruments included in the protocol.

Chronicity Prediction Checklist. Van Riper (1971), after reviewing literature concerned with differentiating between the characteristics of a moment of stuttering and disfluency, created a list of guidelines for differentiating normal from abnormal disfluency. That 1971 listing, as well as the research available to that time, led to the creation of the Cooper Chronicity Prediction Checklist for Stuttering (Cooper, 1973). Relying on data obtained in other investigations (Lankford & Cooper, 1974; McLelland & Cooper, 1978; Riley, 1981), the checklist was subsequently revised and incorporated in the Cooper PFCT-R children's fluency assessment digest.

The revised Chronicity Prediction Checklist consists of 27 questions that the clinician answers with yes or no responses after consultation with the disfluent child's parents and after observations of and interaction with the child. Responses to the questions provide historical data (such as time of onset and family history of stuttering) and information concerning the parents' and child's attitudes toward the stuttering (e.g., do prolongations last longer than one second?). Yes responses are interpreted as predictors of stuttering chronicity, but no individual weighting of individual items for predictive value is attempted. Information is obtained about variables that either have been found to relate to chronicity (e.g., severity) or have been suggested as being related (e.g., self-concept as a stutterer). The Chronicity Prediction Checklist is scored on the basis of the number of yes responses obtained. Two to 6 yes responses are termed as being predictive of recovery, 7 to 15 yes responses as requiring vigilance, and 16–27 yes responses as being predictive of stuttering chronicity. As noted on the Chronicity Prediction Checklist form, the categorization of the scores is based on an interpretation of data reported by McLelland and Cooper (1978) and on clinical observation. The user is cautioned not to make stuttering chronicity judgments solely on the scoring of the checklist.

Parent Assessment. To obtain parent participation in the analysis of the child's fluency, a Parent Assessment inventory is included in the children's version of the fluency assessment digest. This inventory, used either in conjunction with the Chronicity Prediction Checklist or alone, assists the clinician in determining the parents' perceptions of the problem and their attitudes and feelings about it. The single-page, 16-question Parent Assessment inventory determines if parents observe disfluencies, and if they do, what kind of disfluencies are observed, in what conditions, and with what consistency. In addition, the inventory includes items to assist the clinician in determining how the parents respond to the disfluencies and what parental suggestions have proven helpful. At the end of the inventory, parents are asked to make a stuttering severity judgment ranging from mild to severe.

Teacher Assessment. Teachers can be extremely helpful in assessing fluency. To assist clinicians in obtaining that help, the single-page, 13-question Teacher Assessment inventory is included in the children's version of the fluency assessment digest. Similar to the Parent Assessment inventory, it determines if teachers observe disfluencies, and if they do, what kinds are observed, under what conditions, and with what consistency. Teachers are asked if they discuss the disfluencies with the child. Finally, teachers are asked to make a severity judgment ranging from mild to severe.

Fluency Assessment. Although reluctant to make stuttering severity judgments on the basis of stuttering frequency counts, stuttering frequency is a major component of any assessment of stuttering severity. The children's fluency assessment digest includes the determination of stuttering frequency counts while the child is reciting, responding to questions, repeating phrases, reading aloud (if able), identifying pictures, and speaking spontaneously.

Duration of Stuttering. Clinicians, using a stopwatch, are asked to estimate the typical duration of a moment of stuttering during the recorded 2–3 minute segment of child's spontaneous speech, elicited by having the child respond to the picture stories included in the children's fluency assessment digest.

Concomitant Behavior. In this single-page checklist, clinicians are asked to check which of the 32 listed behaviors that frequently accompany the act of stuttering have been observed in the child being evaluated. These behaviors are listed under five categories: posturing, respiratory, facial, syntactic and semantic (judged to be stuttering avoidance behaviors), and vocal. To be checked by the clinician, these behaviors need not occur during every moment of stuttering but should be in the child's current repertoire of concomitant behaviors.

Attitudinal Indicators. This single-page form to assess the child's attitudes toward fluency is omitted with preschool children for whom clinicians judge it to be inappropriate. The form consists of 20 attitudinal statements that are read aloud to the clients. The children are asked if they agree or disagree with the statements. Clinicians are advised to modify or omit statements they feel would not be appropriate for the children with whom they are working. Agreement with a statement indicates the child holds an attitude that may be a problem needing attention. Many mentally retarded stutterers have difficulty in responding to auditorially presented attitudinal statements such as those presented in the Cooper PFCT-R assessment digests. In such situations, clinicians are able to obtain indications of the clients' attitudes through the use of pictures found on the PFCT-R's "Stuttering Attitudes Stimulus Sheets" and the "Speech Situation Discussion Sheets." These blackline story drawings depict various speaking situations to which clients are asked to respond. The drawings are useful both with children and adults, and clinicians find them particularly useful with nonreaders.

Situation Avoidance Reactions. Ten speech situations common to school-age children are listed in this brief secton of the assessment digest. Additional spaces are provided for other situations that might be identified by the child or the clinician. Children are asked to indicate which of these situations they avoid or would prefer to avoid because of their fluency. This section is omitted when the clinician thinks it would be inappropriate for the child being assessed.

Child's Perception of Stuttering Severity. Children are asked in three different ways to indicate how much of a problem they believe their fluency to be. Their responses are placed on a 3-point severity scale.

Clinician Perceptions of Severity. Upon completion of the assessment instrument, clinicians are requested to make 5-point-scale severity judgments on five aspects of the child's fluency: frequency, duration, consistency across speech situations, concomitant behaviors, and handicapping reactive attitudes and feelings.

Adolescent and Adult Fluency Assessment Digest

The "Cooper PFCT-R Assessment Digest and Treatment Plan—Adolescent and Adult Version" consists of a 12-page booklet. The assessment digest portion is 7 pages in length. The first page of the assessment digest contains client identification information and a form for summarizing the assessment data obtained on the following 6 pages. At the bottom of the first page, the clinician, after completing all assessment activities, judges the extent to which the client's fluency problem is socially and vocationally handicapping. On the succeeding 6 pages of the form, the following dimensions of the client's fluency are assessed:

>Frequency of stuttering
>Duration of stuttering Moments
>Situation avoidance reactions
>Concomitant behavior
>Attitudinal indicators of significance of stuttering
>Client perceptions of severity
>Clinician perceptions of severity

Frequency of Stuttering. Stuttering frequency counts are made while the client is reciting, repeating, reading (if able), responding to questions, and speaking spontaneously for 2–3 minutes.

Duration of Stuttering Moments. The clinician, using a stopwatch, estimates the average duration of the client's moments of stuttering during the recorded two to three minutes of spontaneous speech. The spontaneous speech is elicited through topics of conversation suggested to the clinician in the fluency assessment digest.

Situation Avoidance Reactions. On a single page form, 50 common speech situations are listed. The clients are asked to indicate which of the situations they avoid or would prefer to avoid because of their fluency.

Concomitant Behaviors. Similar to the procedure used in the children's version, clinicians are asked to check which of the 32 listed behaviors frequently accompanying the act of stuttering are observed in the client being evaluated.

Attitudes toward Stuttering. Clients are asked whether they agree or disagree with 25 statements concerning stuttering. This inventory is scored by adding the number of statements with which the client agreed.

Agreement with the statements is interpreted as indicating the client's attitude is undesirable with respect to that issue. A significant number of agree responses is interpreted as indicating a significant attitudinal problem on the part of the client.

Client Perceptions of Severity. Similar to the children's version form, except using a 5-point rather than a 3-point scale, the client is asked to judge the severity of the fluency problem by completing three sentences concerning the problem.

Clinician Perceptions of Severity. Identical to the children's version form, clinicians are requested to make 5-point scale severity judgments with respect to the client's stuttering frequency, duration, consistency, concomitant behaviors, and handicapping reactive attitudes and feelings.

THERAPY WITH THE MENTALLY RETARDED STUTTERER

The successful utilization of behavior modification programs with mentally retarded populations in the late 1950s and early 1960s undoubtedly was a major factor in the dramatic proliferation of behavior therapies that continues to this day. It was, and still is, assumed that behaviorally oriented therapy programs are particularly effective and efficient with the mentally retarded because they circumvent dependence on the higher cognitive functioning that is impaired in the mentally retarded. It is no surprise, therefore, to find that most fluency programs for the mentally retarded typically are exclusively behaviorally focused. Frequently, little or no attention is directed to shaping and reinforcing fluency-facilitating attitudes and feelings in the mentally retarded stutterers.

The Therapy Process

The following discussion of therapeutic strategies for the mentally retarded stutterer is based on the *Cooper Personalized Fluency Control Therapy—Revised* program (Cooper & Cooper, 1985), an integrated cognitive and behavioral therapy process. In addition to the assessment protocols described previously, the PFCT-R kit includes a handbook, a 100-page booklet of therapy materials printed to facilitate duplication, and eight therapy game boards. Many of the materials included in the PFCT-R kit are used effectively with nonreading mentally retarded children and adults. While it is understood that adaptations must be made in the manner in which the PFCT-R process is carried out with the mentally retarded stutterer, a summary of the process appears appropriate. It is labeled the STAR Process (Cooper & Cooper, 1985) and is summarized as follows.

Structuring Stage. The clinician assists the client in identifying behaviors occurring during moments of disfluency and behaviors adopted as a result of the disfluencies. The clinician informs the client of the procedures to be followed in the therapeutic process and, with older clients, the rationale for focusing on the client–clinician relationship to facilitate removal of disruptive cognitive processing and, through the resulting therapeutic involvement, to facilitate the client's acquisition of fluency initiating gestures.

Targeting State. The clinician asks the client to begin modifying behaviors identified in the first stage of therapy. The clinician observes client behavioral patterns indicating resistance to change. Having targeted the client's therapy-impeding and -facilitating behavioral and attitudinal patterns, the clinician makes the client aware of these patterns. The goal of the clinician's confrontive behavior is to lead the client into an affectively dynamic helping relationship. The clinician reinforces the client's expressions of feelings in response to the clinician's confrontations. Through shaping of the client's affective responses, the clinician creates a therapeutic milieu conductive to client identification and evaluation of feelings and attitudes pertaining to the modification of the client's fluency problem.

Adjusting Stage. The clinician reinforces client expressions of affect to facilitate client self-evaluation activities and to maintain client commitment to change. The clinician reinforces accurate, self-appreciative, and productive verbalized client cognitions and reinforces behavioral expressions of adequacy. The clinician instructs the client in self-reinforcement procedures for the maintenance and continued enhancement of the individual. Concomitantly, the clinician instructs the client in manipulating speech behaviors in the therapy environment to determine which fluency-initiating gestures (e.g., speech rate change, the easy onset of phonation, or breathing pattern changes) appear most appropriate for the client. The adjusting stage is brought to a close when both the clinician and the client agree that the client has made sufficient adjustments in fluency-related attitudes, feelings, and behavior to begin to strive for the feeling of fluency control in situations outside of the clinic or the home environment.

Regulating Stage. The clinician assists the stutterer in planning and using fluency-initiating gestures in speech situations in which the client is disfluent. The primary goal in this final stage of therapy is the development of the *feeling* of fluency control. Regularly scheduled therapy may be terminated when stutterers *feel* that no matter how difficult the speaking situation may be, they are capable of employing fluency-initiating gestures to alter their level of fluency, hopefully to a level of fluency acceptable to themselves.

Modifying the Process for the Mentally Retarded

Therapy processes such as the one just summarized encompass complex and continuing verbal interchanges between client and clinician concerning feelings and attitudes. Obviously, with clients whose cognitive processes are in any way impaired, shifts in emphases at various stages of the process must occur if the program is to be successful. While it may appear simplistic, the single most useful modification of the process for the mentally retarded relates to reducing the number of abstract concepts the clinician uses in the process. Therapy goals remain the same, while the therapeutic activities are altered to compensate for the mentally retarded client's lack of conceptual and expressive capabilities.

While most inexperienced clinicians have little difficulty in reacting appropriately to the behavior of mentally retarded stutterers, many respond as if the individual is without feelings and attitudes relative to the behavior. This attitude is reinforced when the mentally retarded stutterer, through either an inability or an unwillingness to do so, gives no indication of possessing such feelings and attitudes. One of the major criticisms of the research discussed earlier in this chapter with respect to assessing stuttering in the retarded relates to the lack of effort directed to determining the affective and cognitive responses of the retarded to their disfluencies. Without exception, judgments as to whether the clients were aware of or affected by their stuttering were based on judgments of listeners rather than on any formal attempt to assess the client's feelings and attitudes.

Experience suggests that mentally retarded stutterers, as is the case with most individuals who stutter, are most successful in obtaining and maintaining fluency when they can identify and express their feelings and attitudes about their problem. In many cases this means that the speech–language clinician must initially focus on teaching the client the ''language of fluency'' before expecting the client to make meaningful progress in therapy. The language of fluency, of course, includes the ability to describe fluent and disfluent speech, to talk about feelings and attitudes, and to talk about specific fluency-enhancing behaviors.

Clinicians who are successful with mentally retarded stutterers invariably attribute their success to their clients' ability to express what they are doing different with their speech to facilitate fluency and their commitment to changing their speech. Even with very young clients, conditioning procedures eliciting fluent speech appear to have little lasting effect unless clients are capable of verbalizing the goal of the procedure and their desire to achieve that goal.

Fluency-Initiating Gestures

Cooper (1976) described a set of fluency techniques and labelled them (Fluency-Initiating Gestures) FIGs. To arrive at these FIGs, a mental factor-analysis of all the fluency-enhancing techniques that clients had reported and that had been observed as being useful was completed. In that manner, a list of six adjustments to an individual's manner of speaking was created and titled the *universal FIGs*. They were termed *universal* because each of the FIGs enhances fluency in most stutterers. The author was aware that the resulting techniques certainly were not new and cited literature dating back to the turn of the century describing these procedures (Cooper, 1976).

Nevertheless, the presentation of the techniques in this fashion facilitates the communication of the procedures to the clients pursuing increased fluency. The universal FIGs are defined as follows:

> *Slow speech:* a reduction in the rate of speech (typically involving the equalized prolongation of syllables).
>
> *Loudness control:* a conscious and sustained increase or decrease in vocal intensity.
>
> *Smooth Speech:* a reduction in the frequency of phonatory adjustments in conjunction with the use of light articulatory contacts (plosive and affricate sounds being modified to resemble fricative sounds).
>
> *Syllable stress:* a conscious loudness and pitch variation.
>
> *Deep Breath:* a consciously controlled inhalation prior to the initiation of phonation (typically used in conjunction with easy onset).
>
> *Easy onset:* a gentle superimposition of phonation on a gentle exhalation.

Teaching the FIGs

Fortunately for clinicians working with mentally retarded stutterers, each of the FIGs can be quickly and easily defined and demonstrated.

Using such graphic illustrations as the "FIG Tree," which are provided in the PFCT-R kit, the concept of fluency-initiating gestures is conveyed to the client. Included in the PFCT-R kit are games and pictures that provide clinicians with materials to stimulate the practice of the various FIGs as well as to reinforce the concepts behind the fluency altering activities.

Frequently, mentally retarded stutterers receive the services of speech–language pathologists in environments where group stuttering therapy situations can be arranged. The teaching of FIGs is enhanced significantly when several individuals in the same environment can support each other in their usage. The concept of FIGs lends itself to establishing a spirit of camaraderie in such a situation. In addition, the therapy's end goal of earning the feeling of fluency control can be easily discussed in the group situation. Typically, the concept of the feeling of control is immediately meaningful to at least one member of the group, who can help explain it the others. Following are brief comments about various aspects of teaching FIGs to mentally retarded stutterers. More detailed discussions of various aspects of the teaching of each FIG are included in the PFCT-R Handbook (Cooper & Cooper, 1985).

Effectiveness Varies. The effectiveness of any one of the FIGs in eliciting fluency varies from client to client. A specific FIGs' effectiveness appears related to the primary observable phonatory, respiratory, and articulatory posturings that occur during moments of disfluency. For example, the deep breath FIG is used effectively by the client whose disfluencies occur most frequently when the client is "out of breath" and attempting phonation without an adequate air supply to sustain it. Another example is the client whose articulatory rate during fluent and disfluent speech is abnormally rapid. That client finds the slow speech FIG is most useful in enhancing fluency.

Order of Teaching. Clients may begin with any one of the FIGs, and there is no set order in which FIGs need to be employed. In the exploratory period when the concept of FIGs is introduced, clients may feel more comfortable beginning with, for example, easy onset rather than the slow speech FIG. Clinicians use their own judgment in advising clients on the order in which they should begin to master the motor acts of the various FIGs. In fact, clinicians may find it helpful to have the client focusing on more than one FIG at the same time. Again, these are judgments best left to the discretion of the clinician. Generally, however, clinicians find that beginning with the slow speech FIG is advantageous because of the ease with which it can be communicated, even to the lower functioning clients.

Need for Instrumentation. Devices to monitor or to display the abruptness of the initiation of phonation and instruments such as the delayed auditory feedback mechanism, metronomes, and noise generators can be used effectively in teaching FIGs. However, they are not critical to the process. An audio recorder and a stopwatch are the only equipment needed in using the teaching materials in the PFCT-R. For example, clients are able to gain a feeling for a slower rate of speech through the utilization of a delayed auditory feedback apparatus. However, the feeling of rate control can be achieved with the use of a stopwatch. Similarly, an instrument indicating abrupt changes in phonatory activity may be an efficient means of assisting clients in developing the feeling of control over the easy onset of phonation, but a clinician can serve as a monitor of easy onsets without expensive instruments.

Need for Overlearning. The skills necessary for successfully executing FIGs appear, particularly to the unexperienced, to be simple. As clinicians well know, they are not simple. Frequently, clients, after completing a few practices in the clinical situation on a given FIG, will feel they have mastered it and are reluctant to continue practicing what may be, in fact, a tedious and dull routine. Clinicians, knowing that the client must become a proficient and knowledgeable manipulator of the basic processes of speech in order to develop the feeling of control, do all they can to maintain the client's perseverance in the FIG exercises. For example, long after the child is able to successfully complete a one-second-per-syllable slow speech FIG exercise in therapy, the child will need to continue such exercises. So it is with all the FIG exercises. Clients must continue to practice the basic skills required for each FIG even after they are using the FIGs effectively in stressful speech situations. Unfortunately, as any knowledgeable amateur athlete will testify, exercises in the basics must be continued even after the skills are being used routinely in the athletic event. The lack of perseverance in drilling on the basic skills that underly each FIG may be the single greatest obstacle to stutterers developing and sustaining the feeling of control.

Side Effects of Teaching FIGs. The fact that many disfluent mentally retarded speakers have accompanying problems in articulation, rate of speech, and voice quality, with a resulting loss of intelligibility, was noted in the review of literature. Experience has shown that improvements in all of these aspects of speech may occur as the stutterer begins to adopt fluency-initiating gestures. This is not surprising. As stutterers begin to use such techniques as slow speech, easy onset, or smooth speech, the basic processes of speech are altered. Thus improvements in articulatory behavior and in phonatory behavior are facilitated at the same time the client is focusing on a fluency-enhancing activity.

Disfluency Descriptor Digest. One instrument developed to assist clinicians in determining which FIG or FIGs appear most appropriate for individual clients is the Disfluency Descriptor Digest (Cooper, 1982). This instrument (see Figure 6.1) has been found to be particularly useful with the mentally retarded stutterer. The Disfluency Descriptor Digest is a single page form that includes a list of 20 statements describing behaviors frequently observed in disfluent speech of stutterers. A check mark is placed in the box preceding the statement if the behavior is present in the client's sutttering pattern, even if the behavior described occurs only occasionally. Following the list of 20 behaviors is a table indicating six fluency-enhancing techniques and the numbers of the behavioral statements that appear predictive of the successful utilization of each particular technique. A frequent clinician observation is that this behavioral checklist assists in identifying the characteristics of each stutterer's disfluencies with more precision and, as a result, assists in increasing the client's awareness of vocal adjustments necessary for increased fluency.

Service Delivery Systems

Since the late 1960s, efforts have been made to "deinstitutionalize" our handicapped populations and to place them in the "least restrictive" environment. Thus, mentally retarded individuals of all but the severe and profound classifications are now served in every type of rehabilitative–educative situation. At the same time, recognizing this population's potential for self-support and for making economic as well as humanistic contributions to society, both governmental and private agencies have developed extensive networks of support programs and services for the group. These support systems, as noted previously, have facilitated the delivery of speech–language pathology and audiology services to the mentally retarded. Such services are now frequently provided through the public schools, community rehabilitiation facilities, associations for retarded citizens, hospitals, United Way–supported programs, and "half-way" houses, as well as traditional residential facilities. Obviously, each of these situations provides speech clinicians unique opportunities, as well as problems, in delivering their services.

Group and Individual Therapy. The question as to whether group or individual stuttering therapy with the mentally retarded is more effi-

THE UNIVERSITY OF ALABAMA
DEPARTMENT OF COMMUNICATIVE DISORDERS

PERSONALIZED FLUENCY CONTROL THERAPY
DISFLUENCY DESCRIPTOR DIGEST
For the Identification of
Appropriate Fluency Initiating Gestures

CLIENT _____   FILE NO. _____

CLINICIAN _____   DATE _____

Directions: Below are statements describing behavior frequently observed in the disfluent speech of stutterers. Place a check (✓) in the box preceding the statement if the behavior is present in the client's stuttering pattern even if the behavior described occurs only occasionally.

☐   1.   Disfluencies are characterized by obvious "struggle behavior" in the laryngeal area prior to speech onset.

☐   2.   Frequently the disfluency is characterized by obvious articulatory posturings of the jaw, lips, or tongue prior to the initiation of sound.

☐   3.   Speech appears monotone with abnormally little variation in intensity or pitch.

☐   4.   The onset and the termination of speech sounds in continued speech appears abnormally abrupt.

☐   5.   The breathing pattern for speech appears to be more "clavicular" or "thoracic" than abdominal.

☐   6.   Articulatory movements appear abnormally rapid.

☐   7.   The habitual pitch level appears too high or low for the individual's age, sex, and size.

☐   8.   The voice quality appears "harsh", "husky", or "hoarse".

☐   9.   In general, the rate of speech appears rapid.

☐ 10.   Disfluencies frequently are characterized by rapid and repetitious articulatory movements of the jaw, lips, or tongue.

☐ 11.   During periods of disfluency, the breathing pattern appears asynchronous and disruptive to fluent speech.

☐ 12.   Disfluencies frequently are characterized by fixed articulatory placements of the jaw, lips, or tongue resulting in a complete closure of the vocal tract.

☐ 13.   Disfluencies frequently appear to originate at the level of the larynx with an inability to initate phonation.

☐ 14.   Inhalation prior to the speech attempt appears abnormally rapid.

☐ 15.   Inhalation prior to the speech attempt appears insufficient.

☐ 16.   Inhalation prior to the speech attempt appears abnormally prolonged.

☐ 17.   Speech appears abnormally soft with respect to loudness.

☐ 18.   Disfluencies appear to occur at the end of an exhalation - client appears "out-of-breath."

☐ 19.   Pauses are observed between the cessation of inhalation and the initiation of phonation.

☐ 20.   Speech appears abnormally loud.

Directions: Now place a check before those numbers in the box below that correspond to the statement numbers that you checked above. When finished you might be able to identify more clearly which FIG or FIGs will be most helpful for your client.

FIG: Fluency Initiating Gesture	Numbers of statements above describing behavior modified by the FIG
Slow Speech	☐ 6 ☐ 9 ☐ 10
Smooth Speech	☐ 4 ☐ 8 ☐ 12
Easy Onset	☐ 1 ☐ 2 ☐ 7 ☐ 12 ☐ 13 ☐ 19
Deep Breath	☐ 5 ☐ 7 ☐ 11 ☐ 14 ☐ 15 ☐ 16 ☐ 18
Syllable Stress	☐ 3 ☐ 11 ☐ 12
Loudness Control	☐ 3 ☐ 8 ☐ 17 ☐ 20

E. Cooper, 1981

FIGURE 6.1   Disfluency Descriptor Digest.

cacious appears to be an academic one. A meaningful response to the question, however, is that a combination of both group and individual therapy is most advantageous. In many situations group therapy is not feasible, simply because of the small numbers of stuttering clients involved. This situation is mitigated in some instances by the formation of "communicaton skills" groups, which bring together clients with various types of communicative disorders. Work toward obtaining most, if not all, of the goals and objectives of fluency therapy can be undertaken in such a heterogeneous group. In fact, in many residential settings, speech–language pathologists utilize such communication skills groups as their primary strategy in improving their residents' communicative abilities. Obviously, clinicians in such settings see the clients on an individual basis to determine the nature of the client's communicative disorders, but the intervention program relies predominantly, and apparently successfully, on group work.

Capitalizing on Supportive Personnel. Speech–language pathologists, having determined what behaviors clients need to learn and having set specific therapeutic goals, can maximize their effectiveness through the use of supportive personnel. Many mentally retarded individuals are in education or rehabilitation situations where supportive personnel are employed. Speech clinicians frequently have the opportunity to train such personnel to become "communication aides." These aides can assist the mentally retarded client in carrying out the tedious and repetitious exercises needed to "overlearn" fluency-eliciting gestures. In residential situations, aides under the direction of speech–language pathologists are turning previously unstructured social situations into communicaton skills sessions. Such situations are excellent examples of creative utilization of aides to increase the efficiency and the effectiveness of the communication disorders specialist with the mentally retarded.

SUMMARY

Following a presentation of the definition of mental retardation and classification systems used in its description, the prevalence of stuttering in mentally retarded populations was discussed. The lack of research concerning the nature of stuttering in the mentally retarded was noted. The few published studies addressing the topic were reviewed and summary observations of the implications of these studies were made. The chapter continued, after a discussion of diagnostic considerations and assessment instruments, with a description of therapeutic strategies and a brief description of systems used in bringing these services to the mentally retarded stutterer.

This chapter began with the observation that the study of stuttering in atypical populatons provides the discipline of human communication sciences and disorders with opportunities to better understand stuttering in all populations. After a review of the published studies of stuttering and disfluent behavior in mentally retarded populations, it is apparent our discipline is still on the threshold of exploring those opportunities presented by that atypical population. Undoubtedly, the current research focus on the neurophysiology of stuttering will extend into the 1990s. Such efforts are leading to an increased interest in disfluent mentally retarded populations. With that should follow the development of even more effective intervention programs for the mentally retarded stutterer. The challenge is here. The future is bright.

REFERENCES

Andrews, G., & Harris, M. (1964). *The syndrome of stuttering* (Clinics in Developmental Medicine No. 17). London: Spastics Society Medical Education and Information Unit in Association with William Heinemann Medical Books.
ASHA Committee on Mental Retardation/Developmental Disabilities. (1982). Serving the communicatively handicapped mentally retarded individual. *Asha*, 24(8), 547–553.
Ballard, P. B. (1912). Sinistrality and speech. *Journal of Experimental Pediatrics*, 1, 298–310.
Blackhurst, A. E., & Berdine, W. H. (1981). *An introduction to special education*. Boston: Little, Brown and Company.
Bloodstein, O. (1981). *A handbook on stuttering*. Chicago: National Easter Seal Society.
Boberg, E., Ewart, B., Mason, G., Lindsay, K., & Wynn, S. (1978). Stuttering in the retarded: II. Prevalence of stuttering in EMR and TMR children. *Mental Retardation Bulletin*, 6, 67–76.
Bonfanti, B. H., & Culatta, R. (1977). An analysis of the fluency patterns of institutionalized retarded adults. *Journal of Fluency Disorders*, 2, 117–128.
Brady, W. A., & Hall, D. E. (1976). The prevalence of stuttering among school-age children. *Language, Speech and Hearing Services in the Schools*, 7, 75–81.
Cabanas, R. (1954). Some findings in speech and voice therapy among mentally deficient children. *Folia Phoniatrica*, 6, 34–39.
Chapman, A. H., & Cooper, E. B. (1973). Nature of stuttering in a mentally retarded population. *American Journal of Mental Deficiency*, 78, 153–157.
Cooper, E. B. (1973). The development of a stuttering chronicity prediction checklist for school-age stutterers: A research inventory for clinicians. *Journal of Speech and Hearing Disorders*, 38, 215–223.
Cooper, E. B. *Personalized fluency control therapy*. Austin: Learning Concepts. (1984)
Cooper, E. B. (1982). A disfluency descriptor digest for clinical use. *Journal of Fluency Disorders*, 7, 355–358.
Cooper, E. B. (1984). Personalized fluency control therapy: A status report. In M. Peins

(Ed.), *Contemporary approaches in stuttering therapy* (pp.   ). Boston: Little, Brown and Company.

Cooper, E.B., & Cooper, C. S. (1985). *Cooper personalized fluency control therapy—revised.* Allen: DLM/Teaching Resources.

Daly, D. A. (1977). *Intervention procedures for the young stuttering child.* Paper presented at the annual meeting of the Council for Exceptional Children, Atlanta, GA.

Edson, S. K. (1964). *The incidence of certain types of nonfluencies among a group of institutionalized mongoloid and non-mongoloid children.* Unpublished master's thesis, University of Kansas, Lawrence, KS.

Farmer, A., & Brayton, E. R. (1979). Speech characteristics of fluent and dysfluent Down's syndrome adults. *Folia Phoniatrica, 31,* 284–290.

Gottsleben, R. (1955). The incidence of stuttering in a group of mongoloids. *Training School Bulletin, 51,* 209–218.

Grossman, H. J. (Ed.) (1983). *Classification in mental retardation.* Washington, DC: American Association on Mental Deficiency.

Guitar, B. & Bass, C. (1978). Stuttering therapy: The relation between attitude change and long-term outcome. *Journal of Speech and Hearing Disorders, 43,* 392–400.

Karlin, I. W. & Strazzulla, M. (1952). Speech and Language problems of mentally deficient children. *Journal of Speech and Hearing Disorders. 17,* 286–294.

Keane, V. E. (1970). *An investigation of disfluent speech behaviors in Down's syndrome.* Unpublished master's thesis, University of Oregon, Eugene, OR.

Keane, V. E. (1972). The incidence of speech and language problems in the mentally retarded. *Mental Retardation, 10,* 3–8.

Lankford, S. D., & Cooper, E. B. (1974). Recovery from stuttering as viewed by parents of self-diagnosed recovered stutterers. *Journal of Communication Disorders, 7,* 171–180.

Lerman, J. W., Powers, G. R., & Rigrodsky, S. (1965). Stuttering patterns observed in a sample of mentally retarded individuals. *Training School Bulletin, 62,* 27–32.

Louttit, C. M. & Halls, E. C. (1936). Survey of speech defects among public school children of Indiana. *Journal of Speech Disorders, 1,* 73–80.

Lubman, C. G. (1955). Speech program for severly retarded children. *American Journal of Mental Deficiency, 60,* 297–300.

Mandell, C. J. & Fiscus, E. (1981). *Understanding exceptional people.* New York: West.

Martyn, M. M., Sheehan, J., & Slutz, K. (1969). Incidence of stuttering and other speech disorders among the retarded. *American Journal of Mental Deficiency, 74,* 206–211.

McLelland, J. K., & Cooper, E. B. (1978). Fluency-related behaviors and attitudes of 178 young stutterers. *Journal of Fluency Disorders, 3,* 253–263.

Otto, F. M., & Yairi, E. (1975). An analysis of speech disfluencies in Down's syndrome in normally intelligent subjects. *Journal of Fluency Disorders, 1,* 26–32.

Preus, A. (1973). Stuttering in Down's Syndrome. In Y. LeBrun & R. Hoops (Eds.), *Neurolinguistic approaches to stuttering.* The Hague: Mouton.

Riley, G. D. (1981). *Stuttering prediction instrument for young children.* Tigard, OR: C.C. Publications.

Schaeffer, M. & Shearer, W. (1968). A survey of mentally retarded stutterers. *Mental Retardation, 6,* 44–45.

Schlanger, B. B. (1953a). Speech examination of a group of institutionalized mentally handicapped children. *Journal of Speech and Hearing Disorders, 18.*

Schlanger, B. B. (1953b). Speech measurements of institutionalized mentally handicapped Children. *American Journal of Mental Deficiency, 58,* 114–122.

Schlanger, B. B., & Gottsleben, R. H. (1957). Analysis of speech defects among the institutionalized mentally retarded. *Journal of Speech and Hearing Disorders, 22,* 98–103.

Schubert, O. W. (1966). The incidence rate of stuttering in a matched group of institutionalized mentally retarded. Convention address, American Association of Mental
Deficiency, Chicago.

Sheehan, J., Martyn, M. M., & Kilburn, K. L. (1968). Speech disorders in retardation.
American Journal of Mental Deficiency, 73, 251–256.

Stark, R. (1963), [Unpublished fellowship thesis]. London: College of Speech Therapists.

Tate, M. W. & Cullinan, W. (1962). Measurement of consistency in stuttering. *Journal of
Speech and Hearing Research, 5,* 272–283.

Wohl, M. T. (1951). The incidence of speech defect in the population. *Speech, 15,* 13–14.

Van Riper, C. (1971). *The nature of stuttering.* Englewood Cliffs, N.J.: Prentice-Hall.

Van Riper, C. (1982). *The nature of stuttering.* Englewood Cliffs, N.J.: Prentice-Hall.

Weiss, D. A. (1964). *Cluttering.* Englewood Cliffs, N.J.: Prentice-Hall.

Yairi, E. & Clifton, N. F., Jr. (1972). Dysfluent speech behavior of preschool children, high
school seniors, and geriatric persons. *Journal of Speech and Hearing Research, 15,* 714–
719.

Zisk, P. K. & Bialer, J. (1967). Speech and language problems in mongolism: a review of
the literature. *Journal of Speech and Hearing Disorders, 32,* 228–241.

7

The Clutterer

David A. Daly

Cluttering has been referred to as the orphan in the family of speech–language pathology. Although this intriguing speech disorder has received considerable attention by European clinical researchers, it has enjoyed only sporadic attention in American professional literature. However, renewed interest in "organic" type stuttering (e.g., Kidd, 1980; Liebetrau & Daly, 1981; Moore, 1984; Quinn & Andrews, 1977; Riley, 1983; Rosenbeck, Messert, Collins, & Wertz, 1978; Rosenfield, 1979) should contribute significantly to our understanding of central language disturbances in general and to cluttering in particular.

Through his 1964 text, Weiss made a valiant attempt to acquaint the American speech–language pathologist with cluttering. Luchsinger and Arnold also devoted noteworthy space to cluttering in their 1965 text. During the 1960s, Arnold utilized the journal *Logos* to present a series of articles on cluttering to professionals in the United States (Arnold 1960a,1960b). In 1970, an entire issue of the journal *Folia Phoniatrica* (Volume 22, No. 4–5) was devoted to the elucidation of this puzzling disorder. (All thirteen articles in this special issue were published in tribute to Deso A. Weiss on the occasion of his seventieth birthday).

Dalton and Hardcastle (1977) included a scholarly chapter on cluttering and disfluency of organic origin in their British text. In addition to numerous suggestions for therapeutic intervention, they propose a host of ideas for both basic and applied research projects.

American speech–language pathologists have not, by and large, accepted cluttering as a clinical entity, nor have they incorporated information about cluttering into their clinical decision-making processes.
Although considerable literature on cluttering exists, American authors
treat the problem of cluttering in a most cursory manner. Typically, only
a paragraph or two are devoted to this ill-understood disorder. Many
authors omit any mention of cluttering.

After dealing for more than twenty years with children and adults
who stutter, the author is of the opinion that cluttering is a separate
clinical entity that is intricately related to the problem of stuttering. Quite
definitely, the two disorders frequently occur simultaneously (Freund,
1952; Van Riper, 1971; Weiss, 1964; Wyatt, 1969). It is not yet clear, however, whether one disorder typically precedes the other. Freund (1952)
and Weiss (1950) both contend that stuttering evolves out of cluttering.
Other authors have noted that cluttering occasionally evolves from stuttering.

This chapter introduces the reader to salient features and characteristics of cluttering. Similarities and differences are cataloged and discussed. Strategies for differential diagnosis are highlighted and various
treatment procedures are presented. Two case studies are included for
illustrative purposes.

CLUTTERING DEFINED

Unfortunately, cluttering is no easier to define than stuttering. As is
the case with stuttering, a universally agreed-upon definition has not
been accepted. British speech pathologists have made some progress
towards a uniform definition. Through their College of Speech Therapists they have suggested that in addition to some of the manifestations
of stuttering, cluttering is characterized by an uncontrolled speed of utterance resulting in truncated, dysrhythmic, and incoherent utterances
(see Dalton & Hardcastle, 1977).

Another standard definition has been provided in *Webster's Third International Dictionary* (Gove, 1981); which defines cluttering as "a speech
defect in which phonetic units are dropped, condensed, or otherwise
distorted as a result of overly rapid agitated speech utterance" (p. 431).

Seeman and Novak (1963) analyzed the marked acceleration of the
clutterer's speech tempo. They found that clutterers' speaking becomes
faster and faster within words and within common phrases. They suggested that this intraverbal acceleration of speech was subcortically
caused. Specifically, Seeman and Novak defined cluttering as the pro-

pulsive impulse to speak, expressed in increasing acceleration, leading to irregular, nonpredictable distortion and omission of consonant sounds and occasionally to rapid repetition of syllables (see Wyatt, 1969).

Most clinical investigators agree that excessive speed is one component that defines cluttering. This *tachylalia* (Greek term meaning fast speech) is indeed a frequently observed feature of the disorder. However, Foreschels (1955) reported that only 50% of his objectively defined tachylalia cases could be classified as clutterers. Speed alone is not enough to warrant the label "clutterer." For example, the very rapid speaker in the televised Federal Express commercial could not be classified as a clutterer. Other deficiencies in language development and formulation, articulation, and awareness must be present for such a diagnosis.

It appears that a universal definition for cluttering does not exist. Early contributors (Bakwin & Bakwin, 1952; Froeschels, 1946; Hunt, 1861) as well as more recent clinical researchers (Arnold, 1960a; Langova and Moravek, 1970; Van Riper, 1971; Weiss, 1964) suggest different orientations and definitions. Realizing that most definitions would be too narrow to include all of the many forms that cluttering may take, we are prone to adopt Weiss' (1964) orientation towards a more global disability of central language imbalance. Specifically, his 1964 definition of cluttering is as follows:

> Cluttering is a speech disorder characterized by the clutterer's unawareness of his disorder, by a short attention span, by disturbances in perception, articulation and formulation of speech and often by excessive speed of delivery. It is a disorder of the thought processes preparatory to speech and based on a hereditary disposition. Cluttering is the verbal manifestation of Central Language Imbalance, which affects all channels of communication (e.g., reading, writing, rhythm, and musicality) and behavior in general. (p. 1).

Weiss' notion of a generalized Central Language Imbalance was pervasive. His concept is best illustrated by his figure of a multiple-tipped iceberg with a single base (see Figure 7.1). In Weiss (1950), he posited that the cluttering child's multiple deficiencies share a common pathological basis. Figure 7.1 shows a markedly different theoretical orientation than the single-tipped iceberg that Sheehan (1970) has used to illustrate the overt and covert aspects of stuttering.

Another plausible explanation for the clutterer's generalized disabilities has been offered by de Hirsch (1961, 1970, de Hirsch & Langford, 1950). She maintained that a lack of maturation of the nervous system is the critical etiological factor. Falck (1969) cites the clutterer's inability to integrate as a possible causative factor. He labeled his conceptual framework of cluttering an integrative mechanism disorder. These hy-

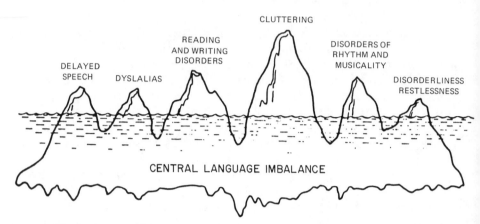

FIGURE 7.1   Weiss' (1964) illustration of multiple, interrelated problems of cluttering with a common base.

potheses are noteworthy; however, clinical experience leads us to support Weiss' notion that cluttering is the manifestation of Central Language Imbalance in the area of verbal utterance (Weiss, 1964). Although Wohl (1970) concurs with Weiss that a language imbalance exists in cluttering, she maintains that the imbalance results from the cluttering and not vice versa. Our present state of knowledge about the etiology of cluttering does not allow us to state with any authority which theoretical framework is correct. An alternative strategy at this juncture may be to describe the various features of cluttering as clearly and precisely as we can.

DESCRIPTION AND CHARACTERISTICS

An author's perceptions of cluttering reflect the basic philosophical orientation of that individual. One writer may portray cluttering as a psychological problem, while another considers it a clumsiness in articulation. Still other authors define cluttering as a deficit in auditory perceptiveness, central language processing, learning disability, and so on. Cluttering represents many different things to many different people.

Obligatory Symptoms

While clutterers may show many different signs and symptoms, Weiss (1964) has argued that only three signs are pathognomonic and essential to the diagnosis. His three obligatory symptoms are an excessive number of repetitions in speech, short attention span and poor concentration, and lack of (complete) awareness of the problem. Weiss lists other cluttering symptoms as faculative (frequently occurring but not mandatory). Surprisingly, he identifies reading disorder as the most common faculative symptom, and not rapid rate of speech (tachylalia), which so many other writers have mentioned. Because some normal speakers speak too rapidly but with perfect order and articulation, Weiss insists that excessive speech rate must be ruled out as the one primary indicator of cluttering (1964).

Of his three obligatory symptoms, only the repetition of one-syllable words or the first syllable of multisyllabic words is easily documented without direct verbal questioning or formal testing. Both the casual and the trained listener will readily note when such repetitions interfere with communication.

The second obligatory symptom, poor concentration and short attention span, was discussed by Gutzmann as early as 1893. Inefficiency or inattentiveness to focus on the details of persons, places, and things interferes with all learning, but, in particular, with the various channels of comprehension and expression of human language. Liebmann (1900), Pearson (1962), and others have drawn attention to the clutterer's inferior auditory attention. In this regard, we have found specific memory-for-sentences tasks (described later) particularly useful in determining the presence or absence of auditory memory deficiencies.

Finally, the clutterer's awareness of his or her "perceived" difficulty in communicating is a particularly crucial obligatory symptom. Weiss' definition lists unawareness as the *first* characteristic feature of this intriguing disorder, and this ordering was not accidental. Bloodstein (1981) likewise stresses the importance of the awareness factor. Specifically, he reports that the clutterer's fluency disruptions are "unaccompanied by fear, anticipation, any sense of difficulty with specific words or sounds or even a detailed awareness of speaking abnormality" (p. 44). We have observed that cluttering children are frequently confused by a listener's inability to understand their speech. Clutterers accept no blame for the communication breakdown, thinking instead that the listener should pay closer attention. Adolescent and adult clutterers are annoyed and often angered by the persistent attempts of teachers or speech–language pathologists to find a problem, when in the clutterers' minds none exists. (The author has treated a number of salesmen who clutter. Their sales managers insisted that treatment be obtained because customers had complained that the salesmen were difficult to understand. Even when therapy was mandatory to maintain employment, some adult clutterers would not take their speech treatment seriously. They preferred to believe that their boss was being "hard-nosed" or unreasonable.)

This genuine lack of awareness of denial is common in cluttering. Freund (1952) suggests the possibility of clutterers' hereditary neurotic dispositions. Obviously, the prognosis is not good for such unaware, unmotivated clients who may be angry about their parents', teachers', or employers' insistence on treatment.

It is easy to understand why unaware clients do not seek treatment. However, clients who are partially aware of their cluttering frequently do not seek professional help either. Therefore, we do not really know how many clutterers actually exist. Although it has been estimated that there may be as many clutterers in the United States as there are stutterers, Weiss (1964) pointed out that our White House surveys (e.g., Anderson et al., 1952) have not even listed cluttering as a category in the breakdown of speech and language disorders. The same omission is true for more recent national surveys of communication disorders (see White House Conference on Children, (1970), and the Healey, Ackerman, Chappell, Perring, & Stormer, 1981, review of the prevalence of communication disorders.

Clinician awareness of the signs and symptoms of cluttering is as important for accurate surveys as the client's awareness. St. Louis and Hinzman (1984) surveyed 152 speech–language pathologists about the problem of cluttering. Among their interesting findings was the high frequency of phrase repetitions in the speech of children whom the clinicians suspected were clutterers and the complete or partial unawareness by the children. Interestingly, St. Louis and Hinzman's data revealed that two-thirds of the responding clinicians reported that they felt inadequately trained to identify and treat children and adults who clutter.

Op't Hof and Uys (1974) agree with Weiss' three obligatory symptoms, but they add one more, namely, a reduced capacity of perception. Op't Hof and Uys maintain that neuropsychological deficiencies in visual–motor and auditory–perceptual abilities constitute a fourth pathognomonic sign. Our work (Daly & Smith, 1979) and that of Tiger, Irvine, and Reis (1980) support the inclusion of this fourth obligatory sign.

Presently we do not know whether there are as many clutterers as there are stutterers. It seems reasonable to speculate that many of the "stutterers" currently receiving treatment are clutterers, or perhaps more accurately, they are clutterer–stutterers. Only more accurate identification procedures and surveys will enable us to arrive at more realistic incidence figures. Demographic studies of cluttering are sorely needed.

Faculative Symptoms

The vast majority of cluttering symptoms have been classified as faculative. Statistical pattern analyses of these often present—but not mandatory—symptoms would most likely prove very enlightening; however, such research remains to be done. Numerous faculative symptoms are briefly described below.

Tachylalia

Most clinical investigators cite excessive speed of delivery as a prominent sign of cluttering. Arnold (1960b) noted the hurried, hasty rate of speech and recommended an objective assessment of the clutterers' precipitious speech velocity. Comparisons with the established word or syllable per minute rates of normal speakers would be relatively easy to make.

Bakwin and Bakwin (1952) noted that with the accelerated rate, most clutterers' words virtually tumbled over one another, making speech difficult to comprehend. Wohl (1970) described this prominent, faculative feature of cluttering as *festinating*, that is, speech that becomes faster and faster as it proceeds. Luchsinger (1963) observed that contraction of longer words was apparent in the speech of clutterers, with the rate of acceleration being proportional to the number of syllables uttered. He identified this alteration of production as an intraverbal acceleration. Clutterers with partial awareness of their problem avoid multisyllabic words and extended discussion. Short responses to questions are common. Seeman (1966) stressed the interverbal acceleration of articulation. Specifically the clutterer shortens or omits the essential pauses between words. Natural pauses and punctuation marks are ignored. Intelligibility is adversely affected.

Rapid speech rates and impulsive speech patterns are common in clutterers. Weiss (1964) points out, however, that many clutterers' speech rates do not exceed the average rates of the normal population. Instead, their speech rates are too fast relative to their own abilities. Weiss maintains that regardless of rate "an individual can be diagnosed a clutterer only when his speech shows signs of faulty integration" (p. 23).

Respiration

Arnold (1960b) contends that "respiratory dysrhythmia is the first cause for the clutterer's jerky and explosive speech" (p. 86). Froeschels (1933) noted over 50 years ago that clutterers who speak in short phrases and sentences tend to inhale more frequently. Luchsinger and Arnold (1965) report that "instead of waiting at punctuation marks, the clutterer jumps in irregular spurts from one group of words to the other" (p. 607).

Whether the uneven, truncated, and sporadic speech of the clutterer is affected more by this faulty breathing than by the jerkiness of delivery is not clear. The decisions to employ respiratory exercises in treating cluttering will need to be made on a case-by-case basis.

Phonation

Luchsinger and Arnold (1965) maintain that most clutterers possess clear voice qualities; however, faulty breathing can have a negative effect on their vocal productions. Speech–language pathologists should be aware that various types of dysphonias are possible in clutterers. Faulty patterns of phonation have been attributed as a cause for speech breaks on stressed vowels (Luchsinger & Arnold, 1965).

Articulation

Clutterers experience a multitude of articulation disturbances, varying from mild dyslalia to congenital dyspraxia. Seeman (1966) likened the clutterer's articulation to dyspraxia, as the errors are not bound to specific sounds or blends. Any given sound or sound combination may be affected. Vowels, syllables, words, and phrases are frequently distorted. In Shepherd's (1960) published phonetic descriptions of cluttered speech, he noted numerous inaccurate and slurred articulatory productions, accompanied by the elision (the omission of unstressed vowels or syllables) and substitution of sounds and words. Luchsinger and Arnold (1965) maintain that the skipping of unstressed syllables and replacement of major word particles with the schwa vowel is an outstanding feature. Frequently, consonant combinations are telescoped into simplified phonemes.

The clutterer's poor articulation may be influenced by concomitant poor motor abilities (deHirsch, 1961), poor concentration (Seeman & Novak, 1963), or a combination of both. The retention of infantile articulatory patterns, especially of the sibilants and /r/ and /l/, has been observed. Shepherd (1960) and Arnold (1960b) note that it is not uncommon for such misarticulations to still occur in adulthood.

Weiss (1964) cites drawling and interjections as another separate faculative symptom. By this he means that clutterers use vowel prolongation as a stalling strategy to help them maintain phonation while searching for the next word. These prolongations and frequent interjections of "filler" syllables such as "ah," "mm," "well," and "you know" represent a form of filibustering. The more relaxed the clutterer is in any given situation, the more frequently he or she uses vowel prolongations and interjections.

Another related articulatory symptom is the vowel stop. Liebmann (1900) contended that stoppage on production of initial vowels, with associated mouth opening, was a decisive symptom important for differential diagnosis. Clutterers, of course, do not develop a subsequent fear of a particular vowel sound, as they remain largely unaware of their breaks in speech flow. Cabanas (1954) found vowel stops and other features of cluttering to be common in mentally retarded children. (See Cooper, Chapter 6, this volume, for specific information on mentally retarded stutterers.)

Monotony and Rhythm

Monotony of speech melody has been attributed to a possible lack of musical sense (Arnold, 1960b; Grewel, 1970; Pearson, 1962; Weiss, 1964). Pearson (1962) found that clutterers performed significantly more poorly on the rhythmic portion of the Drake Musical Aptitude Test. While faulty rhythm and melody may be principle characteristics of clutterers' overall disability, Weiss (1964) contends that their speech is not monotonous in the typical sense of the word. Instead, clutterers continually repeat the same short melodic pattern. Such monotonous speech patterns and the accompanying lack of speech rhythm are among the most readily distinguishable symptoms of cluttering. Curiously, many clutterers cannot keep time with simple rhythmic patterns, such as drum beats.

The ability of clutterers to sing is another area open to thoughtful investigation. Some clutterers reportedly improve when singing aloud; others experience considerable difficulty even *trying* to sing. Arnold (1960b) suggests that a musical test has a proper place in the examination of every clutterer. Luchsinger and Arnold (1965) devote an entire section of their text to the relationship between music and language, but collaborative studies by scholars in both specialties are needed.

Motor Abilities

Cluttering children have been described as clumsy, awkward, and uncoordinated (Bakwin & Bakwin, 1952; Seeman, 1966). Similar to their speech productions, their motor activities are accelerated and hasty. Gestures and facial movements are more lively than in noncluttering children (Freund, 1952). Hyperactivity, impulsiveness, and restlessness are terms frequently seen in clinical reports on clutterers. These behaviors contribute to their social rejection by peers. Some cluttering children constantly move around the room during the evaluation session. If they can remain seated, signs of motor overflow are noted in upper or lower extremeties. We have observed that some cluttering youngsters continue to expound about a topic long after the examiner is satisfied with their response. Occasionally, cluttering children appear to be so "wound-up" that they continue talking aloud to themselves even after the examiner shifts topics or leaves the room. This suggests the possibility of some emotional component.

Another interpretation of such behavior has been offered by Seeman and Novak (1963). The speculate that the clutterer's hyperactivity by day and restlessness even when sleeping suggest submicroscopical lesions of the basal ganglia. While hard neurological symptoms have not been confirmed yet in clutterers, their motor deficiencies (and other symptoms) certainly suggest what Weiss (1964) has referred to as an organic flavor.

Many cluttering children are physically small for their age. Their developmental histories show retardation in the age they were able to sit, stand, walk, and hop (Arnold, 1960a) and in the development of speech and language skills (deHirsch and Langford, 1950; Morley, 1957). Left-handedness is common among clutterers, but the same may be true for stutterers. More careful analysis of developmental data on clutterers and stutterers is needed, such as that reported by Bakwin and Bakwin (1952) and Berry (1938).

Disorganized Thought Processes

The incongruity between the clutterer's speed of thought and the speed of speech is a common theory found throughout the literature. Weiss credits Hippocrates for first hypothesizing that stutterers think faster than they can speak (1964, p. 34). Historically, parents have told their disfluent children to "slow down" and to "stop and think of what they want to say before they say it." While such advice undoubtedly has some merit for all of us, coaching a child to organize his or her thoughts and to plan his or her speech acts carefully may be more applicable to clutterers and clutterer–stutterers than to stutterers.

One of the basic, underlying problems for the clutterer is a lack of clarity of inner formulation of speech. It appears as though clutterers omit some vital step in the preparatory process of formulating speech. Froeschels (1946) investigated different types of imagery in speech and concluded that clutterers do not formulate their speech properly. Weiss' (1950) notion that cluttering is a manifestation of a central language imbalance certainly implicates the brain as a primary contributor to this syndrome. Word-finding problems resembling anomia are common; clutterers suffer from an inability to plan ahead. As Weiss (1967), puts it, "they blank out." Frick (1965) found that teaching young adult stutterers strategies for forming, constructing, and evolving motor plans affected a greater reduction in the severity of their stuttering than was found in a matched group of stutterers who received conventional therapy only. It would be interesting to replicate his study with clutterers and clutterer–stutterers. Future speech–neuropsychological studies will undoubtedly shed much light on clutterers' and stutterers' processing difficulties.

Language Difficulties

The presence of a pervasive language disability in cluttering has been articulated by various authors. Here again, Weiss' concept of a central language imbalance has been most widely discussed. Whether the problem is referred to as a developmental or familial disability, or some other label, authorities appear to be in agreement that the genesis is most likely organic.

In her classic study on the developmental history of stuttering, Berry (1938) noted that "the stutterers were definitely retarded" in both their age of first words and their age of intelligible speech, as compared to nonstuttering children (p. 24). She argued that many stutterers begin life with a defective armanentarium for speech (and, we would add, for language, too). Bloodstein (1958), in his Brooklyn College developmental study, also reported that fully one-third of his stutterers were described by their parents as late talkers who persisted for a relatively long time in baby talk and were difficult to understand. Andrews and Harris (1964) noted that 45% of their group of 9-year-old stutterers were late talkers. De Hirsch and Langford (1950) made the following observation about the stuttering children they treated:

"Many of these children start talking late. . . . Frequently their motor

speech patterns are so poor that their speech is practically unintelligible.
. . . Investigation of the family background of these children frequently
reveals a history of language difficulty" (p. 96).

Bluemel (1957), Van Riper (1971), Gregory and Hill (1980), Daly
(1981b), and others have discovered concurrent language disturbances
among their stuttering clients. In fact, Van Riper (1971) identified a separate "track" of stuttering development for approximately one-fourth
of the youngsters whose developmental history he analyzed. He added
that many of his Track II stutterers could be viewed as clutterers.

More recently, Riley and Riley (1979, 1983) reported on several neu-
rologic components of stuttering that they have been investigating. Their
component model applies directly to the complete cluttering syndrome;
however, we limit discussion to their finding of sentence formulation
difficulties instutterers. Such language problems as word retrieval, word
order difficulties, simplication of sentences, and use of fragmentary
phrases were noted in 30% of the 54 stuttering children they studied.
Their differential treatment programs for stuttering children with different disabilities are most encouraging.

Gregory and Hill (1980) also recommend comprehensive evaluations
and differential treatment for stutterers with various deficiencies. They
reported that 55% of their 52 stutterers needing comprehensive therapy
programs demonstrated word retrieval difficulties. Gregory and Hill recommended specific language-oriented treatment programs, prior to
fluency treatment, for suttterers with such problems.

Such frequent occurrence of language problems (and other concomitant problems) in stutterers leads one to speculate that perhaps
cluttering, or at least cluttering–stuttering, may be a more accurate diagnostic classification for many "stuttering" clients. After all, language
disturbances have been considered an integral part of cluttering for de-
cades. For example, deHirsch and Langford (1950), Luchsinger (1957),
and others noted that many clutterers had a poorly developed sense of
language expression that affected grammar and syntax. Improper use
of verbal conjugation, incorrect sequencing of prepositions, and inappropriate reference by pronouns were common impairments. These features and other symptoms of cluttered speech contribute to the confused
and jumbled verbal output of the clutterer. For example, in their haste,
clutterers transpose sounds, syllables, words, and phrases. Such accidental transpositions of initial sounds and parts of speech have led to
experiences that most speakers would consider extremely embarrassing.
Arnold (1960b) cites several classic transpositions. Two of the more well
known transpositions are "The Lord is a shoving leopard" (loving shepherd) and "Sew her to a sheet" (show her a seat) (p. 90.) Surprisingly,

the unaware clutterer is not unduly concerned about his or her verbal faux pas.

Reading and Writing Deficiencies

As mentioned earlier, Weiss (1964) regards a reading disorder as a most prominent faculative symptom. He maintains that a reading disability may even substitute for a decisive diagnostic sign when other conditions make the diagnosis uncertain. The clutterer's impulsive nature interacts with his or her reading efforts. Typically, clutterers skim sentences and paragraphs quickly, often completely missing several syllables or words. Weiss suggests that clinicians have the presumed clutterer read aloud for several minutes, as reading errors may not become evident until the person relaxes his or her concentration skills. Arnold (1960b) reported that clutterers skip entire lines when reading aloud, often repeat other sections, or insert nonexisting words or phrases. More revealing, perhaps, is the clutterer's poor performance in retelling the story to the examiner. Typically, the story line is not followed, details are elaborated, and the main features are confused or omitted. (Story recall is an important facet of comprehensive evaluation with children and adult suspected of cluttering.)

Spadino (1941) studied the writing characteristics of stuttering children and found only small differences in handwriting between his stuttering and nonstuttering children. With clutterers, however, the differences are significantly more pronounced. Errors in writing reflect the clutterers' poor psychomotor coordination. Roman (1959) described clutterers' "agitographia," or disintegrated writing, as "the hallmark of the clutterer who spills out the written word in head-long haste, clipping letters, omitting syllables, slurring substitutes, transposing words, hence, producing in his almost illegible hand the counterpart of his inarticulate speech" (p. 36).

Spelling errors are evident in clutterers' writings, too. Clutterers do not take the time to write double *t*'s or double *e*'s. Roman (1963) contends that poor spelling represents a separate aspect of the clutterer's general language disability. Luchsinger and Arnold (1965) consider writing and spelling errors in families the sign of a hereditary manifestation of constitutional language disability. Because reading, writing, and spelling disabilities are common in cluttering, assessment procedures to establish the presence or absence of possible deficiencies should be a standard part of any comprehensive assessment battery. (Readers interested in various examples of clutterers' figure-drawings, writing, and spelling errors should review Roman's articles.)

Closely associated with such reading and writing disturbances are sinistrality (left-handedness) and mixed laterality. Luchsinger and Arnold (1965) stress that left-handedness alone does not cause either delayed or disordered language acquisiton in clutterers; however, their reported figures of 20% sinistrality for both male and female clutterers are compelling. Hecaen and de Ajuriaguerra (1964) report that left-handedness varies between 5 and 10% in the general population. The finding that clutterers show at least twice the percentage of sinistrality as the normal population is a significant sign that warrants additional investigation. Previous research cited by Hecaen and deAjuriaguerra (1964, pp. 9–10) show that epileptic and retarded groups also show twice the extent of left-handedness as is found in normal subjects. They recommend several procedures for testing handedness, eyedness, and other areas. We would concur that handedness and laterality are important areas to investigate during the cluttering assessment.

Intelligence and Personality

From the information above the reader may have assumed that the majority of children and adults who clutter are somewhat slow intellectually, or even mildly retarded. Arnold contents that, "Low I.Q. does not belong to the tachyphemia syndrome" (1960b, p. 84). Many clutterers demonstrate superior mathematical and abstract reasoning abilities. They may perform below average in language-oriented and music subtests, but their intellectual abilities are more likely to be average, superior, or brilliant.

Nevertheless, cluttering symptoms are evident in some mentally retarded children, especially those with Down's Syndrome. Cabanas (1954) and Weiss (1964) have commented on the rapid, repetitive, unintelligible speech of some retarded persons. Their happy-go-lucky nature and lack of complete awareness are other substantiating symptoms. While mentally retarded stutterers who are responsive to treatment do indeed exist, we are of the opinion that a sizable proportion of them are, in fact, clutterers. The multitude of cluttering symptoms that do legitimately apply to retarded persons would seem to argue in favor of cluttering as the more appropriate diagnosis.

Before leaving the topic of the clutterer's intellectual capacity, we would like to make two additional points. First, like stuttering, cluttering may affect persons at any level along the intellectual range. Second, clutterers are likely to show superior abilities of exact reasoning. Luchsinger and Arnold (1965) specifically mention their high mathematical–quantitative intelligence (Q-type). Clutterers reportedly favor scientific or concrete professions such as engineering, physics, or accounting.

Writers have expended considerable effort describing personality traits and attitudes of clutterers. Descriptions such as impulsive, untidy, careless, hasty, forgetful, and emotionally unstable are typical (Froeschels, 1946; Gutzmann, 1898; Liebman, 1900). Bakwin and Bakwin (1952) observed that clutterers' accelerated and hasty movements, in walking as well as postural attitudes, may be likened to deviations noted in children with cerebral damage. Clutterers' restlessness and apparent aggressive behavior often contribute the their social rejection by peers. The clumsy, messy, disorganized, inarticulate child easily becomes a social outcast. Adolescents are quick to cite any difference or peculiarities in peers. Thus, the cluttering child may be identified in school as "weird" or "a klutz."

In commenting on adult clutterers, Weiss (1964) suggests that they are typically impatient, superficial, and short tempered. Weiss and other researchers have argued that the Greek orator Demosthenes was actually a clutterer, rather than a stutterer as some have claimed. Demosthenes, Weiss pointed out (p. 53), was called *argans* (the violent).

The preceding generalizations concerning the intelligence and personality of clutterers may be interesting. However, the astute clinician realizes that clutterers are people, and as such, they show considerable variation. Similar to clients with other communicative impairments, each clutterer should be considered as an individual.

Heredity

Arnold (1960a), Weiss (1964), Luchsinger and Arnold (1965), and others maintain that heredity plays a prominent role in most cluttering and that the hereditary factor is stronger in cluttering than in stuttering. Arnold declares that previous and present investigators agree on the genetic basis of cluttering. Cases of familial cluttering, including diagrams of family trees, may be found in the literature; however, as Dalton and Hardcastle (1977) point out, the various theories are based upon authors' clinical observations and personal experiences. The fact is that no pathological anatomic findings have, as yet, been reported to substantiate their claims. Perhaps as cluttering becomes more widely recognized and accepted as a clinical entity, genetic studies (such as those conducted at Yale University by Kenneth Kidd and his colleagues) will delineate specific physiologic signs and symptoms (Kidd, 1980). Even though many clutterers appear neurologically underendowed, hard data substantiating organicity are lacking. The sad-but-true fact is that we now have the knowledge and technology to conduct validation studies. Ironically, the following quote by St. Onge and Calvert is as true today as it was 20 years ago when they described the state of the art in stuttering research. In 1964 they noted,

> Is there a predominately organic stutterer who on careful neurological examination would show many positive signs? The painful fact is that after over two thousand studies we cannot answer these relatively simple questions with a substantial statement of how stutterers distribute themselves either on the psychological or organic side. . . . Investigators seldom trouble to perform the necessary diagnostic refinements. (St. Onge & Calvert, 1964, p. 164).

While substantial progress has been made in the area of stuttering, we would argue that St. Onge and Calvert's statement would still apply to dysrhythmic speakers believed to be clutterers.

EEG Findings

Luchsinger and Landholt (1951) conducted one of the earliest studies of electroencephalographic (EEG) examinations on patients with the diagnosis of cluttering. They reported that 90% of the clutterers they examined showed abnormal EEG's. This unusually high figure strongly supported earlier notions that cluttering was organic in nature.

Moravek and Langova (1962) conducted EEG examinations on a larger group of 177 clutterers and stutterers. Twenty eight or 16%, of the group were clutterers, 53 (30%) were stutterer–clutterers, and 96 (54%) were stutterers. The number of abnormal EEG findings for the cluttering group was 50%. This is an impressive statistic but does not approach the 90% figure reported by Luchsinger and Landhold (1951). Only 15.5% of the stutterers showed pathological EEG findings. Individuals affected both with cluttering and stuttering exhibited pathological findings on the EEG 39% of the time. An additional 17% of the combined group showed atypical findings. In summarizing their results, Moravek and Langova noted that their 50% incidence of EEG abnormalities in the cluttering group sufficiently justified the hypothesis that cluttering represents a disease developing on the basis of an organic central nervous system disturbance. In their 1970 article, the same two authors argue that because clutterers can improve their speech by volitional effort (even if only for short periods of time), the EEG abnormalities must be viewed as coordinate symptoms and not as pathogenetic signs. This shift in interpretations is most puzzling. As in so many areas of cluttering and stuttering, we must continue our research efforts to gain a better understanding of even the most elementary information about these disorders.

In 1964, Langova and Moravek reported the results of a more elaborate study designed to clarify the possibility of an organic basis for cluttering. They compared stuttering and cluttering subjects on EEG tests, on their reactions to delayed auditory feedback (DAF), and on the effects of the drugs chlorpromaxine (CLP), a tranquilizer, and dexfenmetrazine, a stimulant. As they had 2 years earlier, Langova and Moravek reported that 50% of the clutterers showed EEG abnormalities, whereas only 15% of the stutterers did so.

Clutterers' and stutterers' reactions to delayed auditory feedback were quite unexpected. Eighty-nine percent of the clutterers reportedly performed more poorly under conditions of DAF, whereas 92% of the stutterers became more fluent under DAF conditions. Langova and Moravek's observation that clutterers expressed unpleasant feelings when using DAF is most interesting.

In response to the CLP drug, 85% of the clutterers reportedly improved, whereas no effect on the stutterers was observed. Just the opposite occurred with dexfenmentrazine. The speech of all eight clutterers in the experiment deteriorated, while 15 of the 17 stutterers reportedly improved their speech. Essentially, clutterers improved with the tranquilizer and responded poorly to the stimulant. The Langova and Moravek study did not demonstrate conclusively the organicity of all clutterers. Rather, it differentiated certain features by which cluttering and stuttering may be objectively viewed as separate clinical entities.

Summary of Descriptive Features and Characteristics

In this section we have highlighted numerous signs and symptoms believed to be characteristic of cluttering. The section that follows compares and contrasts the disorders of cluttering and stuttering. Before examining those similarities and differences, however, it is instructive to note the many features that cluttering has in common with yet another syndrome, namely, learning disabilities. The impulsive, untidy, inattentive, unaware, underachiever in school, who suffers from specific reading disabilities and oral language disturbances, could easily belong to either category. Writing disabilities and dysrhythmia are common for either group. We support Tiger and her colleagues' (1980) contention that cluttering should be viewed as a complex of learning disabilities. The excessive speech rates, unusual prosodic patterns, and perceptual deficiencies are similar for both groups. Pervasive language disabilities are common core bases of both groups. And, the incidence of both cluttering and learning disabilities is four times higher for males than females (Arnold, 1960b; Cruickshank, Morse, & Johns, 1980; Froeschels, 1946).

Clinicians and teachers may improve their understanding of these disorders if mutually beneficial discussions and collaborative teaching and research ideas are explored. Speech–language pathologists have readily accepted the clinical practice of "staffing" cleft palate and cerebral-palsied clients. We have recommended such intradisciplinary and interdisciplinary staffings for stutterers (Daly, 1984). In view of the multiple problems of clutterers, and the different orientations of various professionals who treat them, we propose that such interdisciplinary discussions are even more obligatory for the cluttering learning-disabled child. Hypothetical professional boundaries must be relaxed if the school-age cluttering child's needs are to be seriously addressed and realistically treated.

COMPARISONS BETWEEN CLUTTERING AND STUTTERING

Considerable effort has been expended to elucidate how stuttering and cluttering are different. Freund (1952), Weiss (1967), Van Riper (1970), and others have summarized salient clinical impressions and experimental findings that may be helpful in differential diagnosis. While many lists contrasting the two disorders may be found in the literature, the 1967 comparative table by Weiss is the most comprehensive. His table (1967, p. 99) is reproduced verbatim in Table 7.1. In examining the various similarities and differences listed for each clinical entity, the reader is reminded that such findings may vary from sample to sample and that differences were generalized from what different authors have interpreted to be typical cases. Considerable variability does exist, and only future objective studies will determine whether certain findings may be viewed as rules or facts about cluttering or as exceptions to the rules.

Interestingly, Table 7.1 focuses on the differences between the two groups. Wingate (1976) suggests that while differences are often of great importance, their relative values frequently do not become clear until commonalities are reasonably well identified and understood. Thus, we would suggest close scrutiny of similarities between samples as well as differences. (In this regard, Rentschler (1984) reported an interesting study exploring commonalities among subgroups of stutterers using neuropsychological assessment.) Whether one elects to explore the sim-

Table 7.1
Weiss' (1967) Comparative Table Showing Various Differences
between Stuttering and Cluttering[a]

	Stuttering	Cluttering
Interpretation	Functional; secondary	Hereditary; primary central
Underlying disturbance	Neurovegetative dys-functional	language imbalance (lack of muturation of CNS mostly absent
Awareness of disorder	Strong	Mostly absent
Speech characteristics		
Specific symptoms	Clonic and tonic inhibition	Hesitation, repetition (without inhibition)
Rate of delivery	Rather slow	Mostly quick
Sentence structure	Mostly correct	Often incorrect
Fear of specific sounds	Present	Absent
Hightened attention (superiors)	Worse	Better
Relaxed attention	Better	Worse
Foreign language	Worse	Better
Gesturing	Stiff, inhibited	Broad, uninhibited
Reading aloud		
Well-known text	Better	Worse
Unknown text	Worse	Better
Writing chracteristics	Compressed; high-pressure strokes	Loose, disorderly
School performance	Good to superior	Underachiever
Psychological attitudes	Embarrassed, inhibited	Carefree, sociable
	Painstaking, compulsive	Impatient, impulsive
	Grudge-bearer	Easily forgetting
	Penetrating	Superficial
Experimental responses:		
Alcohol	Better	Worse
Lee-effect	Better	Worse
EEG	Borderline normal	Often deviant
Chlorpromazine	Worse	Better
Dexfenmetrazine	Better	Worse
Course	Fluctuating; spontaneous Improvements and relapses	Persistent
Therapy	Attention should be diverted from details; psychotherapy	Concentration on details
Prognosis	Depends on emotional adjustment	Depends on acquiring concentration

[a]Reproduced from Weiss (1967, p. 99).

ilarities or contrast the differences, many potentially fruitful topics for scientific inquiry may be gleaned from Table 7.1. Various images of stutterers and clutterers have been perpetuated in both professional and lay literature. Through research, these images or clinical impressions will be either substantiated or refuted.

Weiss (1950, 1967) presented another useful scheme to depict the interrelationship between cluttering and stuttering and to illustrate how the entire fluency-disordered group may be divided. In this model Weiss (1967) portrays one-sixth of the total group as pure clutterers and another one-sixth as pure stutterers. The remaining 66% he contends are clutterer–stutterers. This mixed group contains individuals who are afflicted with various features of both disorders. Some cases have predominate symptoms of cluttering, while in others symptoms of stuttering predominate. This mixed group may have inherited a common disposition to both conditions (West, Ansberry, & Carr, 1957).

Langova and Moravek (1964) reported that 16% of their 177 subjects were clutterers, 54% were stutterers, and the remaining 30% were clutterer–stutterers. Van Riper's (1971) tracking system for differentiating developmental stuttering patterns specified 14% and 25% respectively for his two samples of possible cluttering-like youngsters. It is not clear whether or not these "clutterers" are merely a subtype of stuttering (Freeman, 1982; Van Riper, 1970). Weiss, (1964) has insisted that all stutterers are basically clutterers. Daly (1981b) and Preus (1981) reported that 24% and 18% of their subjects, respectively, fit into Van Riper's Track II subgroup.

Since the mid-1970s we have carefully scrutinized each fluency client seen in our clinical program. Comprehensive diagnostic tests have been administered and results catalogued (see Daly, 1981b, for protocol and preliminary findings). Our findings show that the number of clients we diagnosed as pure clutterers was quite small (less than 5%). The number of pure stutterers seen was approximately 55%. A sizable number of clients (40%) were classified into the cluttering–stuttering group. Our proportions are similar to those of Dalton and Hardcastle (1977), who report that they have worked with a large number of clutterer–stutterers, but only a few pure clutterers. Our mixed group would have been even larger had we included stutterers with one or two concomitant disabilities. However, just because a stuttering youngster also had reading difficulty or an articulation problem, he or she did not qualify for the cluttering–stuttering group (many clients in our pure stuttering group did indeed have other problems). Like Blood and Sieder (1981), we were surprised to find so few stutterers with no other problems. Apparently, the old adage that children who stutter are no different from nonstuttering children, except for the fact that they stutter, is not as true as many of us were led to believe.

ASSESSMENT PROCEDURES

This past decade has witnessed the publication of several excellent clinical perspectives on assessment procedures for clients with fluency disorders (see Conture, 1982; Gregory & Hill, 1980; Hood, 1978; Riley & Riley, 1983; Shine, 1980; Williams, 1978). Rather than reiterating various standard procedures here (e.g., rate of speech, type of disfluency, analyzing possible maintenance factors), this section highlights a number of procedures that may have merit when cluttering is suspected.

Of course, a thorough case history of the client, including questions about speaking characteristics of family members, is invaluable. When a negative response is received to questions regarding the possibility of cluttering and stuttering disorders in relatives, we have followed Weiss' (1964) suggestion of asking additional questions about any hasty speakers or unusually rapid talkers.

This tactful approach is usually more descriptive for most parents, and possibly less threatening. Asking parents to bring their child's baby book to the evaluation also is helpful in verifying motoric and speech and language developmental milestone information. During the interview, we probe for information about restlessness, hyperactivity, inattentiveness, and academic performance. We want to know such things as strong and weak areas in school (particularly mathematics, reading, and writing) and overall academic performance. If conducted, we request copies of psychological and social worker evaluations. We inquire about the child's medical history. In particular, we are interested in any perinatal complications, use of sedatives or tranquilizers and the presence of allergies. Interestingly, we have found that 40% of the cluttering–stuttering children we have treated over the last 4 years have allergies—Whether or not children in Michigan have an unusually high incidence of allergies we do not know—and many parents have commented that when the allergic reactions occur, stuttering also exacerbates. Since allergies do affect the respiratory abilities of many children, we believe they are worth noting.

Parents are asked to check appropriate identifying items on an adjective checklist, including characteristics such as withdrawn, extroverted, immature, friendly, disorganized, unconcerned, and clumsy. Parents' responses serve as leads for more in-depth questions. Cooper's (1973) chronicity predictive checklist for school-age stutterers is utilized to organize our interview and obtain specific information in the shortest time possible. The parental interview is extremely important and should not be discounted. Whenever possible, one clinician interviews the parents while another begins the assessment with the child.

We closely observe the inspiratory and expiratory breathing patterns of the client, not only during speech acts, but during rest and oral reading tasks as well. Recall that respiratory dysrhythmia is most common in cluttering. Inappropriate breath groups, jerky breathing, and speaking on reserve air should be noted. We also monitor the person's vocal characteristics to rule out any related or concomitant problem with phonation or resonation.

A detailed articulatory assessment is mandatory! Our studies (Daly, 1982) have revealed that 52% of the stuttering children we have followed either showed concurrent articulation problems or had received prior treatment for such errors. Conture (1982) report a 66% prevalence figure for his stuttering clients, while Riley & Riley (1983) report 41%. Needless to say, the co-occurrence is high. Precise transcriptions of the client's speech will determine whether the suspected clutterer exhibits a "garden-variety" lisp or distoration or whether vowel stops, interverbal acceleration, elision, and skipping of unstressed vowels or syllables, or other unusual errors are common features of his or her speech. Repeated analyses of recorded speech and oral reading samples are typically necessary for accurate assessment.

Elicited imitation procedures and prompting increasingly longer words (such as *please, pleasing, and pleasingly,* and *zip, zipper, zippering*) are useful techniques to obtain samples of multisyllabic words. Many clutterers have experienced so much negative feedback regarding the lack of intelligibility of their speech when they attempt polysyllabic words that they omit them from their vocabularies.

The majority of clutterers we have seen are compulsive talkers. Obtaining an adequate speech sample to assess tachylalia is not a problem. Keeping them on a topic is the problem. Occasionally, we encounter a possible clutterer with low verbal output. The creative ability of the clinician to elicit an adequate speech sample is tested. Our stimulation strategies are dependent upon the age and reading ability of the client, of course, but unless clinicians obtain samples of verbal output, diagnosis is futile. In difficult cases we revert to simpler tasks, such as identifying pictures, simple oral reading, or sentence imitation.

We have found our memory for unrelated sentences task (Daly, 1981a; Daly, Ostriecher, Jonassen, & Darnton, 1981) particularly useful in this regard. Immediate auditory memory abilities for connected speech are determined through sentence imitation, and clients generally relax and are more cooperative after this simple task. Thirty-eight percent of our stuttering clients scored 2 years or more below normal levels on this task (Daly & Smith, 1979). Riley and Riley's (1983) data indicate that 37% of their stuttering subjects demonstrated attending disorders. Inasmuch as concentration and attending constitute an obligatory symptom of cluttering, sufficient time should be spent evaluating such abilities. Auditory comprehension, memory, and processing skills should be assessed with various tests and subtests familiar to the examiner.

Many language tests are available for assessing various aspects of comprehension and performance. Rather than list tests and measures we prefer, we suggest that clinical judgment be exercised when selecting age-appropriate language tests. We would add, however, that oral reading abilities need to be investigated. We intentionally select reading material that is at least 1 year behind the person's expected reading level. We recommend tape recording at least 3 to 5 minutes of their oral reading for later analysis. Omissions, insertions, and increased rate are often not observed until after a short period of guarded reading.

Another useful dimension to explore is storytelling. For younger children we employ Goldman and Fristoe's (1969) sounds-in-sentences stories. Even with pictures, continuity is difficult for clutterers. For adolescents and adults, Wechsler's (1945) standardized stories for immediate and delayed recall are utilized. The individual's ability to recall relevant points and to follow the story line are documented and contrasted to norms.

Motoric responses can be very informative. Our observations begin when the client first walks into the office. Unusaul gait, posture, and facial movements are noted. The presence or absence of motor overflow in the form of foot movements or finger tapping and twitching facial musculature are documented. Figure drawing and writing responses are obtained. Children are asked to draw a figure of a person and then to write (or print) their name and a simple sentence like "The grass is green."

Hand preference is noted and eye preference is assessed. Hand–eye coordination and neuropsychological processes are tested with Smith's (1973) Symbol Digit Modalities Test (See Smith, (1975), for complete description). Basically, this symbol-substitution test measures the ability to process numbers for simple geometric figures. The Symbol Digit Modalities Test is reportedly sensitive to the presence of organic cerebral impairment. Because both written and oral scores are provided and because both of the subtests take less than 5 minutes to administer, we give it routinely to all clients.

The Purdue Pegboard Test is routinely administered to all clients. This measure of manual dexterity is reportedly a very efficient method of screening for brain damage and detecting laterality of a lesion (see Lezak, 1976, for a description of the test and Costa, Vaughan, Levita, & Farber, 1963, for clinical applications). Daly and Smith (1979) reported that 24% of their "functional" stutterers performed in the definitely subnormal range on the Purdue Pegboard, whereas 38% of their stutterers with additional learning disabilities showed subnormal performances.

Pearson (1962) and Weiss (1964) cite poor rhythm in speech as one of the more noticeable symptoms. They contend that clutterers have difficulty in perceiving and reproducing rhythmic beats. We ask each disfluent youngster to sing "Twinkle, Twinkle, Little Star" and to reproduce the melody for the chant, "Johnny's got a girlfriend." Some clutterers find such rhythmic tasks most difficult. Presently, we are exploring stutterers' and clutterers' responses to Froseth's (1979) Kinesthetic Response to Rhythm in Music Test. Stutterers' and clutterers' abilities to respond to a series of tempo beats and to the steady rhythmical sense of their own internal pulses also are being investigated.

Whenever possible, each client is tested with the Michigan Neuropsychological battery (see Smith, 1975). We conducted studies (Daly & Smith, 1976, 1979; Smith & Daly, 1980) to differentiate stutterers according to the presence or absence of associated neuropsychological deficiencies. Findings indicated three or more signs of neuropsychological deficiencies in 43% of our presumedly functional stuttering group ($N = 74$) and in 93% of the stutterers with identified learning disabilities ($N = 14$). Rentschler (1984) reported an interesting comparative study using various neuropsychological procedures with stutterers. Collaborative research between the disciplines of speech–language pathology and neuropsychology to elucidate brain–behavior relationships in stutterers and clutterers is felt to be critically important.

The extent to which the clutterer is aware of or concerned about his or her communication handicap and his or her attitudes and feelings about the problem are diagnostically significant. The best way to determine a clutterer's awareness or concern is to ask. Thompson (1983) has published a useful 18-item attitudinal interview for school-age children who stutter. Erickson (1969) and Woolf (1967) have designed attitudinal instruments for older children and adults. We have found Woolf's Perceptions of Stuttering Inventory (PSI) particularly helpful for diagnostic purposes and for measurement of treatment effectiveness (Daly & Darnton, 1976). Modification of attitudes is essential to carryover (Guitar & Bass, 1978). Many clutterers, however, are annoyed with questions about stuttering, as they do not perceive themselves to have a problem. To obtain an estimate of their level of awareness we use a modified PSI that we designed some years ago. The Perceptions of Communication Inventory (Daly, Oaks, Breen, & Mishler, 1981) consists of the same 60 items as the PSI, except that the words *speech* or *speaking difficulty* have been substituted for the word *stuttering*. Thus, the altered inventory does not mention stuttering in its title or items. High school and college age normal-speaking students checked an average of 10 or fewer items as characteristic of their speech. Clutterers check an average of 5 or 6 items on this attitudinal measure. Most clutterers are unaware or partially unaware of their speech difficulty. We recommend some form of formal assessment of this dimension.

This section has highlighted selective procedures for identifying and assessing cluttering. Some strategies were based on normative data, while others were conceptualized empirically. There is much to be learned about cluttering. The literature is more extensive than many may have believed. Knowledge of published literature will guide researchers and clinicians in their future decisions. But much, perhaps most, of the reported findings on cluttering need to be verified. *Research* means to search again, and we must replicate many studies and create new ones. Like detectives searching for clues, we must probe further whenever we suspect a discrepancy between what we observe with a patient and what's been written about them. To quote my colleague, Aaron Smith (personal communication, 1980), "When the behaviors and characteristics we observe in our patients do not agree with those described for such cases in the book, throw away the book. The patient can't be wrong." Clinicians must follow their clinical hunches when assessing individuals presumed to be clutterers.

The final section of this chapter reviews various treatment strategies believed to be beneficial to clutterers. Two case studies are included for illustrative purposes.

THERAPEUTIC CONSIDERATIONS

Numerous anecdotal comments and suggestions for treating cluttering are found in the literature. Surprisingly, not one controlled, systematic report on therapeutic efficacy could be found. Prognostic statements range from the historical generalization that cluttering is virtually untreatable to Froeschels' (1946) assertion that every case treated with his procedures could be "cured within three to six months" (p. 33). Froeschels designed a pictorial phonetic script showing how the lips, teeth, and tongue should be positioned for enunciating specific sounds. He also recommended that his cluttering patients transcribe reading passages into his phonetic alphabet several times each day. Froeschels also stressed lipreading exercises to assist clutterers in focusing on the precise movements necessary for detailed articulation. Such conscious awareness of sound formation had the side benefit of slowing the clutterer down while simultaneously helping him to bring his fast speech tempo in line with his motoric production.

Weiss (1960, 1964) agreed that treatment for cluttering should emphasize concentration on the sharply defined details of speech production. When excessive speed of delivery was one of the presenting symptoms, Weiss recommended a syllabization procedure. Specifically, the clutterer would slowly pronounce each syllable, giving each syllable equal duration. (Interestingly, a similar "droning" effect results from use of a delayed auditory feedback machine. We have found it advantageous to drone volitionally with our clients early in therapy when they are required to drone at different rates.) Syllabization and droning generally heightens the client's awareness to his or her tactile and kinesthetic feedback systems, and they point out that fluency and rate are features of speech over which he or she can exercise some control. To improve clutterers' poor rhythmic sense, Weiss favored rhythmical finger-tapping to every slowly pronounced syllable. Other strategies Weiss advocated are simultaneous oral reading, shadowing, and pronouncing each syllable while writing it. Volitional accentuation of each stressed syllable was strongly advised. Bradford (1963) concurs with accentuations but insists that each clutterer also finger-tap the accented syllables. Tiger and her colleagues (1980) report success in using a metronome to train more fluent and intelligible speech.

Other recommended methods include underlining the final consonants of words (Bradford, 1963), as they tend to be slurred the most, and looking up proper accents in the dictionary (Weiss, 1960). To counteract the clutterer's monotonous or stereotyped rhythmic pattern, Arnold (1960b) suggested recognition and duplication of simple, then more complex, rhythmic beats.

Weiss (1964) suggested counting backward to increase concentration. He maintains that even well-educated clutterers will show difficulty counting backward by 3's or 4's. He also stresses the memorization of poems, story repetition, and joke-telling to combat the clutterer's chronic problem of fluctuating attention. Weiss (1964) warns that transfer is difficult unless several sessions are spent on story sequencing. Training on silent sentence formulation before verbalization typically is needed. Weiss contends that coaching clutterers to visualize the written words or phrase before pronouncing them is quite helpful.

Luchsinger and Arnold (1965) contend that if education in grammar, syntax, and composition are needed, clinicians may follow activities suggested for aphasic patients. Activities are suggested for the improvement of faulty patterns of breathing, phonation, articulation, projection, and cluttered handwriting. Luchsinger and Arnold also propose some training on basic appreciation and expression of music, rhythm, and dance, as well as an orientation to social poise. They maintain that many clutterers require such reeducation to meet the expectations of society.

Interested readers are referred to Bradford's (1963) excellent review of other therapeutic procedures for clutterers. She makes two points that are emphasized here. First, many clutterers need to be taught that silence is as much a part of effective communication as sound. Second, self-monitoring skills are absolutely critical for accurate evaluations of one's own performance. To quote Bradford, "Only when the patient begins to evaluate the correctness or incorrectness of his production does the new speech habit become, actually, a part of his speech pattern" (1963, p. 61). Her statement is as powerful today as it was in 1963, for self-monitoring plays such an essential role in our effective treatment procedures. After all, one of the clinician's primary tasks is to help the clutterer develop a fuller awareness of his or her speech pattern and an effective means for consciously monitoring his or her own speech.

We have experienced encouraging results with clutterers by employing a modification of Shames and Florance's (1980) Stutter-Free Speech Program. Their procedures stress the identification and deliberate practice of highly specific speech targets. Their emphasis on slow, smooth speech initiations and continuous phonation, first with delayed feedback and later without it, provides the clutterer with concrete, verifiable components of the speech act that can also be monitored. Moreover, Shames and Florance's use of a visible hand signal serves as an efficient physical and mental reminder to the client that he or she is to do something different when beginning each speech act. Their self-evaluation forms and speech contract sheets enable the clutterer to become more and more self-reliant in self-instruction, self-monitoring, self-evaluation, and self-consequation. Because Shames and Florance's evaluation forms and contract sheets allow the clinician to ascertain whether the clutterer or stutterer is experiencing difficulty with any of the targets, we strongly recommend their use (Daly, Carter, & Simon, 1983). Bandura (1977), Kanfer (1974), Stewart (1974), and Florance and Shames (1980) have emphasized that a client's motivation is positively affected when specific goal-setting and self-evaluative procedures are utilized. Such self-monitoring activities are exceedingly helpful to cluttering clients.

To our surprise, most of our cluttering–stuttering clients have not experienced undue difficulty in using the delayed feedback machine, as did Langova and Moravek's (1964) patients. However, when off the machine, some find volitionally droning at different rates especially troublesome. Several sessions of clinician modeling are frequently needed. We employ numerous lists of specifically prepared phrases and sentences at this stage of treatment. For example, short sentences containing nonplosive sounds are used first. Later, longer sentences that contain plosives are introduced. This strategy seems to facilitate the clutterer's correct production of the continuous-phonation speech target. Added benefits of using specifically written sentences are that (1) the clinician knows precisely what words the client is supposed to say, and (2) breath support can be monitored by controlling the length of the stimulus material. Of course, speaking with constant phonation also forces the client to talk at a slower rate.

Occasionally, a client encounters unusual difficulty in comprehending the continuous phonation target. He or she persists in producing choppy speech even after various verbal explanations and modeling. In such cases Conture's (1982) analogy of a garden hose, faucet, and nozzle has proven helpful. Two of our mentally retarded clutterer–stutterers grasped the continuous phonation concept only after we demonstrated, with water in the sink, how water could be released either in bursts or spurts or in a smooth, continuous flow. Only then did they completely understand our explanation of the smooth, constant voicing of speech. Once understood, however, these retarded youngsters moved ahead in the program. We have found it best with mentally retarded clients and younger clutterers with associated problems to teach one speech task at a time. Cooper's (1979) fluency-initiating gestures have been utilized successfully in this regard. Success with clutterers, and other clients, comes not only from the client's hard work, but from clear and concrete explanations and demonstrations by clinicians. Because most clutterers exhibit problems attending and concentrating, we suggest making explanations as clear and brief as possible.

Associated problems in such areas as language, oral coordination, articulation, memory, reading, and writing are common in cluttering. Whether to treat the various disorders individually or simultaneously is most likely a decision that can best be made on a case-by-case basis. As mentioned earlier, Riley and Riley (1980, 1983) and Gregory and Hill (1980) have reported success in treating some problems simultaneously. For them, language therapy, syllable training, memory-enhancing activities, articulation work, and so on may be integrated concurrently. For younger clients who have short attention spans, changing activities within a treatment session may be advantageous. Shine (1980) provides many suggestions for keeping younger clients motivated in therapy. For older clutterers, however, we have found it more advantageous to deal with one issue at a time.

Clinical reports (e.g., deHirsch & Langford, 1950; Van Riper, 1971) indicate that clutterers or stutterers with other problems do require more therapy than clients who only stutter. Tiger et al. (1980) reported significant improvement for their clutterer following 9 months of remediation 3 hours per week. Daly's (1982) stutterers with concomitant articulation problems did make progress after 6 weeks of intensive treatment, but when compared to stutterers without other problems, they made the smallest gains. Clutterers do indeed make progress, but usually at a slower rate than stutterers. Because many school-age clutterers are receiving remedial help from other school specialists (e.g., in reading, memory, and writing), we have found it most productive to focus initially on the dimensions of rate and fluency. Clinicians must be involved in the education–remediation plan. Clutterers can be helped and the speech–language pathologist must play a prominent role in their remediation.

CASE STUDIES

The two case studies that follow illustrate many signs and symptoms of cluttering. It should be noted, however, that neither client represents a "pure clutterer"; rather, both were judged to be clutterer–stutterers.

Case 1. Jeffrey, a 9-year, 7-month-old fourth grader, was referred to our program for a stuttering problem. His mother reported that he had been a little slow in starting to talk and that strangers had difficulty understanding him. The father was an engineer and the mother taught music at a nearby junior college. Two older siblings were in high school. Jeffrey's mother indicated that no one else in the family had any speech or language problem. She spoke very rapidly. Upon questioning she did volunteer that many of her students frequently asked her to repeat assignments, indicating that she talked too fast.

Jeffrey's mother reported that the family first noticed his "stuttering" when he was about 4 years of age. She commented that he seemed almost driven to talk. The kindergarten teacher commented on his rapid rate, and since then he had received several poor reports from teachers about his reading and language-arts skills.

At the age of 9 Jeffrey displayed an unusually strong interest in the family's computer. He was beginning to write simple programs and preferred to work with the computer after school rather than play outside with friends. He successfully resisted his mother's persistent efforts to teach him to play the piano.

Initial examination indicated a very rapid (machine gun–like) style of speech delivery, with the end of his sentences trailing off to a mumble. Inconsistent articulation errors were noted, as well as an inattentiveness and jerkiness of response. Testing with our memory for unrelated sentences task and subtests of the Illinois Test of Psycholinguistic Abilities (Kirk, McCarthy, & Kirk, 1968) revealed auditory memory deficiencies. Jeffrey's oral coordination abilities, however, were within normal limits. His draw-a-person figure was immature and his handwriting was jerky. Although his classmates were using cursive writing, he preferred to print; but even his printing was largely illegible.

Jeffrey's appearance impressed us the most. Both parents were impeccably dressed, but he was just the opposite. His shirt tail was hanging out in back, his shoes were untied, and his hair was uncombed. The first thing he did upon entering the examining room was to remove his shoes. He had difficulty sitting still in therapy.

The Stutter-Free Speech Program (Shames & Florance, 1980) was used with Jeffrey, as his very rapid rate and multiple repetitions were the two most disturbing features of his speech. Although he originally did not want to wear the headset to the delayed feedback machine, Jeffrey was persuaded to cooperate. Immediately upon removing the headset, his speech would revert back to his original machine gun–like rapid rate. Several sessions were used to train Jeffrey and his mother to model our slow, easy, drone-type speech. An evaluation form was designed to provide a visual record on which—either mother or son—could indicate the other's success in maintaining a drone (cotinuous phonation at a slow rate). Daily practice periods were scheduled for Jeffrey and his mother, and the evaluation forms were consistently used. After about 2 weeks of practice Jeffrey's speech rate was under stimulus control. He could volitionally employ controlled speech rates with either his mother or the clinician. Shames and Florance's (1980) "let go" speech target was introduced without too much difficulty. Initially, Jeffrey reverted back to his rapid rate at the point in a sentence where he was to change from a controlled slower rate to a normal rate. Here again, extra therapy time was needed to teach Jeffrey and his mother normal speech rates. Stickers and points for special privileges were successful in maintaining his interest throughout this process. "Secret" hand signals (e.g., pressing index finger to thumb) also proved to be especially motivating for Jeffrey. He slowly began to integrate use of his signal with other family members and in school. His speech became increasingly more fluent and his intelligibility improved.

Jeffrey received treatment three times per week for the first month, then twice a week for 6 additional months. Weekly therapy was continued thereafter. In total his program lasted about 18 months. He is now fluent and the family is very pleased with his progress.

A recent discussion with his mother revealed that Jeffrey was receiving extra help from specialists in school. He goes to remedial reading classes twice a week and also receives help with his handwriting. His teacher is working with the mother to improve his grammatical abilities. Mathematics continues to be a strong area for Jeff, and he still spends more time working with the computer than playing with peers.

Case 2. Kurt, a 46-year-old engineer, contacted us for help with his "stuttering." He felt that his speech might be interfering with his career as a sales representative. Previously, he had regarded his "problem" as a minor inconvenience. He recalled having therapy in elementary school for articulation and language problems. He also stated that he was teased as a child for not being very well coordinated. Two factors persuaded him to seek help at this time. First, his boss mentioned that improved speech would make him more valuable to the company. Second, he had noticed that his two sons were beginning to repeat syllables and words like he did. He traveled much of the week but was becoming more aware of his influence with his sons during the weekends. Lately, he found himself talking less and less to them for fear that they might imitate him. Testing revealed sound and syllable repetitions at the beginning of sentences, followed by a very rapid speech rate. Kurt stated that he was talking less in sales meetings and at business social functions. He checked 21 items on the Perceptions of Stuttering Inventory as characteristics of his speech; most items checked were in the avoidance category.

Because of his travel schedule, treatments were scheduled at different times each week. One session might be held at 8:00 in the morning and another at 8:00 in the evening. Two sessions were held each week, and Kurt was very conscientious about attending.

The Stutter-Free Program was followed (Shames & Florance, 1980). Kurt responded quickly to the delayed feedback–volitional droning part of treatment. He suggested making a personal practice tape, including samples of his speech at various delay levels, for use on his business trips. After the first four sessions he reported some carryover of fluency. By the end of the third week he observed that he was maintaining improved fluency for about 24 hours after each session. Kurt used Shames and Florance's self-evaluation forms whenever possible each day to monitor his speech. In the evenings, he reviewed his practice tape. He was diligent about learning to shift smoothly from monitored to unmonitored speech. He practiced with coworkers and strangers, and his speech contract assignment sheets reflected his perseverance. He reported practicing aloud in his car each morning while on his way to work. Kurt viewed these practice sessions as warm-up exercises similar to those a runner uses to loosen up. Within 24 sessions he was fluent in all situations.

During one of our periodic maintenance sessions, Kurt announced that he had been promoted to a vice-president's position within the company. The president had informed him that they had been considering him for some time but did not feel his speech would hold up under the pressures of the job. His speech improvement had been observed, and they now felt confident he could handle the various responsibilities of the position. Kurt also commented that he was spending more time with his boys, going on camping trips and thoroughly enjoying their interactions.

A telephone call made 2 years after the termination of treatment revealed that Kurt's improvement had been maintained. He commented that he had been given additional responsibilities within the company and that he occasionally used his warm-up practice activities before an important presentation.

Not all clients possess the ability or the perseverance to pursue each phase of treatment with Kurt's enthusiasm. He was truly an unusual case, but he is included here to illustrate how cluttering may evolve into stuttering and, also, to show what is possible when motivated clients are introduced to therapy procedures that address their needs.

SUMMARY

Like stuttering, cluttering has been viewed as an incomplete puzzle—a puzzle with many interlocking pieces, many of which we do not yet fully comprehend. Cluttering, on one hand, seems to be closely interrelated with the problem of stuttering. And yet, on the other hand, it seems more appropriate to view cluttering as a separate clinical entity. For some cases, Weiss' concept of a central language imbalance appears to be the most accurate diagnosis. For others, underlying disturbances of prosody, dyspraxia, or aphasia seem to provide more correct explanations of the conditions. We have much to learn about the syndrome or combinations of symptoms called cluttering. Is cluttering really more organic in nature than stuttering? or Do the two conditions reflect opposite ends of a virtual continuum? Future basic and applied research studies will eventually answer these and other questions. But clutterers require our best efforts now. Fortunately, the literature is replete with suggestions for treating clutterers. Comparative studies are needed to demonstrate which procedures are most effective. To compare and contrast various procedures objectively it will become increasingly important for clinicians to document and catalog relevant information such as previous treatments attempted, length of treatment, client attendance, and cooperation of family members. Through such efforts, patterns may emerge that will begin to explain why some clients benefit from remediation, while others do not. Careful record keeping may also identify which features of the clutterer's problems are most effectively treated first, second, and so forth. Different sequences of treatment may emerge for clutterers with different combinations of symptoms.

The clinical speech–language pathologist currently approaches the problem of cluttering with more questions than answers. Three questions that we find particularly intriguing are (1) Do some clutterers spontaneously recover from their impairments the way many stutterers reportedly do? (2) Will some clinically significant deficiencies persist (as

Weiss, 1964; Tiger et al; 1980; and others maintain) even after measure-able gains are achieved in some areas? and (3) Is cluttering the "mother load" of stuttering? or stated differently, Does stuttering evolve from cluttering or vice versa?

These questions, and others, need more careful scrutiny by our scholars and clinical investigators. Few disorders offer such opportunities to explore how so many modalities of communication are interrelated. It is our hope that this chapter has triggered a desire to learn more about this perplexing disorder and that it will encourage readers to utilize their research and clinical skills to help individuals who suffer from this condition.

REFERENCES

Anderson, V. A., Kopp, G. A., Mase, D. J., Schnell, H., Shover, J., Wolfe, W. G., & Johnson, W. (1952). ASHA committee on the Mid-century White House Conference. *Journal of Speech and Hearing Disorders, 17,* 129–137.

Andrws, G., & Harris, M. (1964). *The syndrome of stuttering.* London: Heinemann Medical Books.

Arnold, G. E. (1960a). Studies in tachyphemia: I. Present concepts of etiologic factors. *Logos, 3,* 25–45.

Arnold, G. E. (1960b). Studies in tachyphemia: III. Signs and symptoms. *Logos, 3,* 82–95.

Bakwin, R. M. & Bakwin, H. (1952). Cluttering. *Journal of Pediatrics, 40,* 393–396.

Bandura, A. (1977). Self-efficacy: Toward a unifying theory of behavioral change. *Psychological Review, 84,* 191–215.

Berry, M. F. (1938). The developmental history of stuttering children. *Journal of Pediatrics, 12,* 209–217.

Blood, G. W. and Seider, R. (1981). The concomitant problems of young stutterers. *Journal of Speech and Hearing Disorders, 46,* 31–33.

Bloodstein, O. (1958). Stuttering as an anticipating sturggle reaction. In J. Eisenson (Ed.), *Stuttering: A symposium.* New York: Harper and Row.

Bloodstein, O. (1981). *A handbook on stuttering.* Chicago: Easter Seal Society

Bluemel, C. S. (1957). *The riddle of stuttering.* Dansville, IL: Interstate Publishing Company.

Bradford, D. (1963). Studies in tachyphemia: VII. A framework of therapeusis for articulation therapy with tachyphemia and/or general language disability. *Logos, 6,* 59–65.

Cabanas, R. (1954). Some findings in speech and voice therapy among mentally deficient children. *Folia Phoniatrica, 6,* 34–37.

Conture, E. G. (1982). *Stutering.* Englewood Cliffs, N. J.: Prentice-Hall.

Cooper, E. B. (1973). The development of a stuttering chronicity predictive checklist: A preliminary report. *Journal of Speech and Hearing Disorders, 38,* 215–223.

Cooper, E. B. (1979). Intervention procedures for the young stutterer. In H. H. Gregory (Ed.), *Controversies about stuttering therapy.* Baltimore: University Park Press.

Costa, L. D., Vaughan, G. H., Levita, E., & Farber, N. (1963). Purdue Pegboard as a predictor of the presence and laterality of cerebral lesions. *Journal of Consulting Psychology, 27,* 133–137.

Cruickshank, W. M., Morse, W. C., & Johns, J. S. (1980). *Learning disabilities: The struggle from adolescence toward adulthood.* Syracuse, NY: Syracuse University Press.

Dalton, P., & Hardcastle, W. J. (1977). *Disorders of fluency and their effects on communication.* London: Elsevier North-Holland.

Daly, D. A. (1981a). *An investigation of immediate auditory skills in "functional" stutterers.* Paper presented at the annual meeting of the International Neuropsychological Society, Atlanta.

Daly, D. A. (1981b). Differentiation of stuttering subgroups with Van Riper's developmental tracks: A preliminary study. *Journal of the National Student Speech-Language Hearing Association, 9,* 89–101.

Daly, D. A. (1982). *Considerations for treating stutterers with and without concomitant articulation disorders.* Paper presented at the 58th annual convention of the American Speech-Language-Hearing Association, Toronto.

Daly, D. A. (1984). Treatment of the young chronic stutterer: Managing stuttering. In R. F. Curlee & W. H. Perkins (Eds.), *Nature and treatment of stuttering: New directons.* San Diego: College-Hill.

Daly, D. A., Carter, D., and Simon, C. A. (1983). *Effects of nonintensive stutter-free speech therapy with stuttering children.* Paper presented at the 59th Annual Convention of the American Speech-Language-Hearing Association, Cincinnati.

Daly, D. A., & Darnton, S. W. (1976). *Intensive fluency shaping and attitudinal therapy with stutterers: A follow-up study.* Paper presented at the 52nd Annual Convention of the American Speech and Hearing Association, Houston.

Daly, D. A., Oakes, K., Breen, K., & Mishler, C. (1981). *Perception of Stuttering Inventory: Norms for adolescent stutterers and nonstutterers.* Paper presented at the 57th Annual Convention of the American Speech-Language-Hearing Association, Los Angeles.

Daly, D. A., Ostreicher, H., Jonassen, S., & Darnton, S. W. (1981). *Memory for unrelated sentences: A normative study of 480 children.* Paper presented at the annual meeting of the International Neuropsychological Society, Atlanta.

Daly, D. A., and Smith, A. (1976). *Neuropsychological differentiation in 45 "functional stutterers."* Paper presented at the 52nd Annual Convention of the American Speech and Hearing Association Convention, Chicago.

Daly, D. A., & Smith, A. (1979). *Neuropsychological comparisons of "functional," "organic," and learning disabled stutterers.* Paper presented at the Annual Convention of the International Neuropsychological Society, New York.

de Hirsch, K. (1961) Studies in tachyphemia: IV. Diagnosis of developmental language disorders. *Logos, 4,* 3–9.

de Hirsch, K. (1970). Stuttering and Cluttering: Developmental aspects of dysrhythmic speech. *Folia Phoniatrica, 22,* 311–324.

de Hirsch, K., & Langford, W. S. (1950). Clinical note on stuttering and cluttering in young children. *Pediatrics, 5,* 934–940.

Erickson, R. L. (1969). Assessing communication attitudes among stutterers. *Journal of Speech and Hearing Research, 12,* 711–724.

Falck, F. J. (1969). *Stuttering: Learned and unlearned.* Springfield, IL: Thomas.

Florance, C. L., & Shames, G. H. (1980). Stuttering treatment: Issues in transfer and maintenance. In W. Perkins (Ed.), *Strategies in stuttering therapy: Seminars in speech language hearing, 1,* 375–388.

Froseth, J. O. (1979). *MLR Test of Kinesthetic Response to Rhythm in Music Test.* Chicago: GIA.

Freeman, F. J. (1982). Stuttering. In N. J. Lass, L. V. McReynolds, J. L. Northern, & D. E. Yoder (Eds.), *Speech, Language, and Hearing, Vol. 2.* Philadelphia: Saunders.

Freund, H. (1952). Studies in the interrelationship between stuttering and cluttering. *Folia Phoniatrica, 4,* 146–168.

Frick, J. V. (1965). *Evaluation of motor planning techniques for the treatment of stuttering.* U. S. Department of Health, Education, and Welfare, Office of Education Research Grant Final Report.

Froeschels, E. (1933). *Speech therapy.* Boston: Expression Company.

Froeschels, E. (1946). Clutteirng. *Journal of Speech Disorders, 11,* 31–36.

Froeschels, E. (1955). Contribution to the relationship between stuttering and cluttering. *Logopaedic en Phoniatrie, 4,* 1–6.

Goldman, R., & Fristoe, M. (1969). *Goldman–Fristoe Test of Articulation.* Circle, Pines, MN: American Guidance Service.

Gregory, H. H., & Hill, D. (1980). Stuttering therapy for children. In W. H. Perkins (Ed.), *Seminars in Speech, Language, and Hearing.* New York: Thieme-Stratton.

Grewel, F. (1970). Cluttering and its problems. *Folia Phoniatrica, 22,* 301–310.

Guitar, B., & Bass, C. 1978. Stuttering therapy: The relation between attitude change and long-term outcome. *Journal of Speech and Hearing Disorders, 43,* 392–400.

Gutzmann, H., Sr. (1898). *Lectures on speech disturbances.* Berlin: Fischer.

Healey, W. C., Ackerman, B. L., Chappell, C. R., Perrin, K. L., & Stormer, J. 1981. *The prevalence of communication disorders: A review of the literature.* Rockville, MD: American Speech–Language–Hearing Association.

Hecaen, H., & de Ajuriaguerra, J. (1964). *Left handedness: Manual superiority and cerebral dominance.* New York: Grune and Stratton.

Hood, S. B. (1978). The assessment of fluency disorders. In S. Singh & J. Lynch (Eds.), *Diagnostic procedures in hearing language, and hearing.* Baltimore: University Park Press.

Hunt, J. (1861). Reprinted 1967. *Stammering and stuttering: Their nature and treatment.* New York: Hafner.

Kanfer, F. (1974). The many faces of self-control or behavior modification changes its focus. In R. Stuart (Ed.), *Behavioral self-management strategies, technique and outcome.* New York: Brunner/Mazel Publishers.

Kidd, K. K. (1980). Genetic models of stuttering. *Journal of Fluency Disorders 5,* 187–202.

Kirk, S. A., McCarthy, J. J., & Kirk, W. D. (1968). *Illinois Test of Psycholinguistic Abilities.* Urbana, IL: University of Illinois Press.

Langova, J. and Moravek, M. (1964). Some results of experimental examinations among stutterers and clutterers. *Folia Phoniatrica, 16,* 290–296.

Langova, J. and Moravek, M. (1970). Some problems of cluttering. *Folia Phoniatrica, 22,* 325–336.

Lezak, M. D. (1976). *Neuropsychological assessment.* New York: Oxford University Press.

Liebetrau, R. M., & Daly, D. A. (1981). Auditory processing and perceptual abilities of "organic" and "functional" stutterers. *Journal of Fluency Disorders, 6,* 219–231.

Liebmann, A. (1900). *Vorlesungen ueber Sprachstoerungen: Heft 4. Poltern (Paraphrasia praeceps).* Berlin: Oscar Coblentz Verlag.

Luchsinger, R. (1957). Phonetics and pathology. In L. Kaiser (Ed.), *Manual of phonetics.* Amsterdam: North-Holland Publishing Company.

Luchsinger, R. (1963). *Poltern.* Berlin-Charlottenburg: Manhold Verlag.

Luchsinger, R., & Arnold, G. E. (1965). *Voice-speech-language, clinical communicology: Its physiology and pathology.* Belmont, CA: Wadsworth.

Luchsinger, R., & Landolt, H. (1951). Elektroencephalographische untersuchungen bei stotterern mit und ohne poltererkomponente. *Folia Phoniatrica, 3,* 135–150.

Moore, W. H. (1984). Central nervous system characteristics of stutterers. In R. F. Curlee & W. H. Perkins (Eds.), *Nature and treatment of stuttering: New directions.* San Diego: College-Hill.

Moravek, M., & Langova, J. (1962). Some electrophysiological findings among stutterers and clutterers. *Folia Phoniatria, 14,* 305–316.

Morley, M. E. (1957). *The development and disorders of speech in childhood*. Edinburgh: Livingstone.

Op't Hof, J., & Uys, I. C. (1974). A clinical delineation of tachyphemia (cluttering). *South Africa Medical Journal, 10,* 1624–1628.

Pearson, L. (1962). Studies in tachyphemia: V. Rhythm and dysrhythmia in cluttering associated with congential language disability. *Logos, 5,* 51–59.

Preus, A. (1981). *Attempts at identifying subgroups of stutterers*. Oslo, Norway: University of Oslo Press.

Quinn, P. T., & Andrews, G. (1977). Neurological stuttering—A clinical entity? *Journal of Neurology, Neurosurgery, and Psychiatry, 40,* 699–701.

Rentschler, G. J. (1984). Effects of subgrouping in stuttering research. *Journal of Fluency Disorders, 9,* 207–211.

Riley, G., & Riley, J. (1979). A component model for diagnosing and treating children who stutter. *Journal of Fluency Disorders, 4,* 279–293.

Riley, G., & Riley, J. (1980). Motoric and linguistic variables among children who stutter: A factor analysis. *Journal of Speech and Hearing Disorders, 45,* 504–514.

Riley, G., & Riley, J. (1983). Evaluation as a basis for intervention. In D. Prins & R. J. Ingram (Eds.), *Treatment of stuttering in early childhood*. San Diego: College-Hill.

Riley, J. (1983). *A causal-comparative study of psychological behaviors in stutterers and nonstutterers who exhibit organic factors*. Unpublished doctoral dissertation, California Graduate Institute, Los Angeles.

Roman, K. G. (1959). Handwriting and speech. *Logos, 2,* 29–39.

Roman, K. G. (1963). Studies in tachyphemia: VI. The interrelationship of oraphologic and oral aspects of language behavior. *Logos, 6,* 41–58.

Rosenbek, J. C., Messert, B., Collins, M., & Wertz, R. (1978). Stuttering following brain damage. *Brain and Language, 6,* 82–96.

Rosenfield, D. B. (1979). Cerebral dominance and stuttering. *Journal of Fluency Disorders, 5,* 171–186.

Seeman, M. (1966). Speech pathology in Czechoslovakia. In R. W. Rieber & R. S. Brubaker (Eds.), *Speech pathology: An international study of the science*. Philadelphia: Lippincott.

Seeman, M., & Novak, A. (1963). Ueber clie Motorik bei Polterern. *Folia Phoniatrica, 15,* 170–176.

Shames, G. H., & Florance, C. L. (1980). *Stutter-free speech: A goal for therapy*. Columbus: Merrill.

Sheehan, J. G. (1970). *Stuttering: Research and therapy*. New York: Harper & Row.

Sheperd, G. (1960). Studies in tachyphemia: II. Phonetic description of cluttered speech. *Logos, 3,* 73–81.

Shine, R. (1980). Direct management of the beginning stutterer. In W. Perkins (Ed.), *Strategies in stuttering therapy: Seminars in speech, language and hearing*. New York: Thieme-Stratton.

Smith, A. (1973). *Symbol digit modalities test*. Los Angeles: Western Psychological Services.

Smith, A. (1975). Neuropsychological testing in neurological disorders. In W. J. Friedlander (Ed.), *Advances in neurology,* (Vol. 7). New York: Raven.

Smith, A., & Daly, D. A. (1980). *Neuropsychological assessment: Implications for treatment of aphasic and stuttering clients*. Miniseminar presented at the 56th Annual Convention of the American Speech–Language–Hearing Association, Detroit.

Spadino, E. J. (1941). *Writing and laterality characteristics of stuttering children*. New York: Teachers College Press.

Stewart, R. (1974). *Behavioral self-management strategies, technique and outcome*. New York: Brunner/Mazel Publishers.

St. Louis, K. O. and Hinzman, A. R. (1984). Personal communication.

192

DAVID A. DALY

St. Onge, K. R., and Calvert, J. J. (1964). Stuttering research. *Quarterly Journal of Speech,* 50, 159–165.

Thompson, J. (1983). *Assessment of fluency in school-age children.* Danville, IL: Interstate Printer and Publishers.

Tiger, R. J., Irvine, T. L., & Reis, R. P. (1980). Cluttering as a complex of learning disabilities. *Language, Speech, and Hearing Services in Schools, 11,* 3–14.

Van Riper, C. (1970). Stuttering and Cluttering: The differential diagnosis. *Folia Phoniatrica,* 22, 347–353.

Van Riper, C. (1971). *The nature of stuttering.* Englewood Cliffs, NJ: Prentice-Hall.

Gove, P. B. (Ed.). (1981). *Webster's Third New International Dictionary.* Springfield, MA: Merriam.

Wechsler, D. (1945). A standardized memory scale for clinical use. *Journal of Psychology,* 19, 87–95.

Weiss, D. A. (1950). The relationship between cluttering and stuttering. *Folia Phoniatrica,* 2, 252–262.

Weiss, D. A. (1960). Therapy for cluttering. *Folia Phoniatrica, 12,* 216–223.

Weiss, D. A. (1964). *Cluttering.* Englewood Cliffs, NJ: Prentice-Hall.

Weiss, D. A. (1967). Similarities and differences between cluttering and stuttering. *Folia Phoniatrica, 19,* 98–104.

West, R., Ansberry, M., & Carr, A. (1957). *The rehabilitation of speech.* (3rd ed.). New York: Harper and Row.

White House Conference on Children. (1970). *Profiles of children.* Washington, DC: U. S. Government Printing Office.

Williams, D. E. (1978). Differential diagnosis of disorders of fluency. In F. L. Darley & D. C. Spriestersbach, (Eds.), *Diagnostic methods in speech pathology.* New York: Harper & Row.

Wingate, M. E. (1976). *Stuttering: Theory and treatment.* New York: Irvington.

Wohl, M. T. (1970). The treatment of non-fluent utterance—a behavioral approach. *British Journal of Disorders of Communication, 5,* 66–76.

Woolf, G. (1967). The assessment of stuttering as struggle, avoidance, and expectancy. *British Journal of Disorders of Communication, 2,* 158–177.

Wyatt, G. L. (1969). *Language learning and communication disorders in children.* New York: The Free Press.

8

Diagnosis and Management of Neurogenic Stuttering in Adults

Nancy Helm-Estabrooks

INTRODUCTION

According to the World Health Organization, stuttering consists of "disorders in the rhythm of speech in which the individual knows precisely what he wishes to say but at the time is unable to say it because of an involuntary, repetitive, prolongation or cessation of a sound" (*Manual of the International Statistical Classification of Diseases, Injuries, & Causes of Death*, 1977). Stuttering is most often a developmental phenomenon, that is, one that appears as a child learns to produce language. Sometimes, however, stuttering occurs in adults who have no childhood history of speech disorders. Often this so-called acquired stuttering is associated with a neurological event such as stroke. In these cases, because the etiology is known, the stuttering may be safely referred to as *neurogenic stuttering*. Neurogenic stuttering is not a unitary disorder anymore than aphasia is a unitary disorder. Just as there are varieties of aphasia that are based in part on the location or site of brain damage, so there are varieties of neurogenic stuttering that may be associated with specific loci of brain damage or involvement. It is of more than academic interest to identify the form of neurogenic stuttering manifested by an individual. Knowledge of the form will influence decisions regarding treatment. For example, in a 1978 study, Helm, Butler, and Benson identified two broad forms of neurogenic stuttering: persistent neurogenic stuttering and transient neurogenic stuttering. While both are associated with more than a single brain lesion, the persistent variety was associated with bilateral damage and continued for years of patient follow-up. The transient variety, which lasted only a few days or months, was associated with multiple lesions of *one* cerebral hemisphere. The treatment of these two varieties, of course, will differ. For patients with transient stuttering the treatment may be merely supportive: assuring the patient that he or she is likely to regain fluency in a spontaneous way and by means of this assurance, reducing any anxiety that may inhibit the natural recovery process. The patient with persistent stuttering will be managed differently, and that management will depend, in part, on the specific etiology and concomitant deficits. Perhaps the best way to explain this philosophy of approach is to review the various forms of neurogenic stuttering that have been identified thus far, to illustrate these varieties with case studies, and to describe some therapeutic techniques for managing these cases. This is the approach taken here.

VARIETIES OF NEUROGENIC STUTTERING

Neurogenic stuttering is most frequently reported to occur in persons with no childhood history of stuttering, although a few reports describe recurrence or worsening of childhood stuttering with brain damage.

Neurogenic stuttering in adults can have one of many etiological causes. It has been described in association with stroke, head trauma, progressive diseases such as Parkinson's disease, supranuclear palsy, brain tumor, Alzheimer's disease, and dialysis dementia, and with the use of certain drugs.

Neurogenic Stuttering Associated with Stroke

Strokes have many mechanisms: thrombosis (occlusion of a blood vessel), embolus (occlusion of a blood vessel by material from a more proximal point in the circulation) or hemorrhage (rupture of a blood vessel). Strokes may be large, in the territory of major vessels, or small. Small strokes (lacunes) usually are caused by chronic high blood pressure. Earlier descriptions of neurogenic stuttering attempt to link it to aphasia (Luchsinger & Arnold, 1965). In these descriptions the stuttering is viewed as one aspect of the aphasic syndrome or as a psychological reaction to the aphasia. Stuttering or stuttering-like behaviors have been described in association with amnestic aphasia (Arend, Handzel, & Weiss, 1962), Broca's aphasia (Trost, 1971), apraxia of speech (Canter, 1971), conduction aphasia (Farmer, 1975) and Wernicke's aphasia (Helm, Butler, & Benson, 1978). Helm et al. also describe stuttering in stroke patients who are not aphasic, as do Rosenbek, Messert, Collins, and Wertz (1978) and Mazzucchi, Moretti, Carpeggiani, Parma, and Paini (1981). For these cases there must be an explanation that does not depend upon aphasia as a mechanism. While it is not the intent of this chapter to provide theoretical models for neurogenic stuttering, it is clear that differential diagnosis of the neurogenic stutterer is necessary in order for optimal management to take place. This examination may consist of a speech–language evaluation, as well as a neurological and neuropsychological examination. Depending upon the nature of the brain damage, the patient with neurogenic stuttering may be more or less likely to have aphasia or other disruptions of higher cortical functions. This likelihood is discussed separately for each form of neurogenic stuttering, beginning with that due to stroke.

Strokes involving the left, or language-dominant, hemisphere are likely to produce aphasia if the damage occurs in the primary cortical language areas or neuronal pathways to and from these areas (for a fuller description see Albert, Goodglass, Helm, Rubens, & Alexander, 1981).

Depending upon which language area is involved, the patient may have difficulty understanding the spoken word as well as problems with verbal formulation. For patients with severe aphasia the stuttering component may be of no concern, but for patients with milder aphasia the stuttering may be a frustrating inhibitor of their verbal expression. Successful management of aphasic patients who stutter, therefore, may depend upon the nature and extent of the language problem. The first step in the therapeutic process is to administer a thorough aphasia test such as the Boston Diagnostic Aphasia Examination (BDAE; Goodglass & Kaplan, 1972b), in order to delineate the patient's language strengths and weaknesses. If one finds, for example, that the patient comprehends the written word better than the spoken word, then the clinician may reinforce oral directions with written directions. During the aphasia exam one also must look for evidence that the patient has word retrieval capacities that are inhibited by the stuttering. To help determine this, the patient's capacity for *written* language formulation must be examined. To restate this point: It is important to differentiate faulty word retrieval (aphasia) from faulty motor speech production (stuttering) in patients who, to some degree, may have both of these problems. For example, if an aphasic patient who seems to stutter in conversation is asked to identify a picture of a Key (BDAE, Confrontation Naming Subtest) and says in an effortless way, "k-k-k-key," then one might assume that the patient retrieved the label correctly but has a motor speech problem. If the patient blocks on that word saying; "k-k-," then one might ask him or her to *write* the name. If he or she is able to do this successfully, then one might assume that the problem is not one of word retrieval. If, however, the patient is unable to either say or write the word, then one cannot assume that stuttering was to blame for the failure to say the word. The two cases described below serve to illustrate the importance of differential diagnosis of the stroke patient with stuttering-like symptoms.

A 62-year-old man, who was originally left-handed but forced to change, was referred to the Boston Veterans Administration Medical Center for evaluation of a speech problem that had persisted for 1 year following a cerebral infarct. His childhood history was positive for stuttering, which occurred around the time he was hospitalized at age 5 for diphtheria and subsided at around age 8 with the help of "elocution lessons." In subsequent years, until his stroke, he was a highly fluent individual who was an amateur actor and a salesman. In addition to the speech problem, the stroke also caused swallowing problems (dysphagia), transient right arm and leg weakness (hemiparesis), and right hemisensory deficit. He reported two instances of "blackouts" for which he was hospitalized during the previous decade. He was under treatment for hypertension and hypothyroidism.

Conversational speech was characterized chiefly by repetition of syllables and short words and by sound prolongations, for example, "be-be-be, because" "until-til," and "I was, I was, I was . . . " Repetitions were dysrhythmic and both clonic and tonic in nature. He frequently attempted to avoid dysfluencies by pausing and restarting phrases.

The *Boston Diagnostic Aphasia Examination* (Goodglass & Kaplan, 1972b) was administered and showed normal articulation, grammatical form, and substantive/functor word ratio despite the stuttering. There were no paraphasic errors. Subtests of auditory comprehension, naming, reading, and writing were within normal limits. In addition, apraxia testing showed no evidence of either bucco/facial/lingual apraxia or limb apraxia.

Neuropsychological tests such as the Wechsler Adult Intelligence Scale (Wechsler, 1955) and the Raven Progressive Matrices (Raven, 1960) were administered. Visual analogies were solved better than verbal analogies, but on the whole, performance was in the bright, normal range.

Thus, although this patient had suffered "at the least" a left hemisphere stroke, aphasia testing offered good evidence that his dysfluency was not the product of a word-retrieval disorder. The stuttering could be treated as a motor speech problem uncomplicated by aphasia. For other patients aphasia is an important consideration in the overall clinical picture. A case of stuttering with aphasia is described below.

A 54-year-old man with a history of high blood pressure and carotid artery disease was seen by the speech pathology department 2 weeks after the onset of right hemiparesis and aphasia. At this time his spontaneous speech was hypophonic and well articulated with frequent 4-word utterances and occasional 5–6-word phrases. Grammatical constructions were limited generally to simple declaratives. He tended not to initiate speech and often responded to questioning by repeating all or parts of the examiner's questions. He produced some paraphasias (particularly real-word substitutions) in running speech, and he had obvious difficulty in retrieving and producing substantive words.

Auditory comprehension was significantly impaired for both conversation and formal BDAE testing (an overall Z score of −1.0 standard deviation for four subtests). Series speech was good, as was repetition of words and high probability sentences. Naming, however, was severely impaired for all semantic categories except letters. Reading comprehension and writing also were significantly compromised. A CT scan showed a small left frontal lesion and deep temporal lobe involvement that spared Wernicke's area. The patient entered a course of aphasia therapy and notable gains were made during the next 6 weeks. As language skills improved, however, the patient developed a stuttering problem characterized by repetitions of initial phonemes and prolongation of vowels. At the same time his verbal agility, as measured by his ability to rapidly repeat words such as *mama, fifty-fifty,* and *caterpillar,* began to deteriorate. He now earned only half the possible points on this task for which he had previously earned full credit. Stuttering did not occur on series speech and repetition, but it did occur on naming and oral reading tasks. Despite the stuttering problem, naming of every kind tested by the BDAE had improved significantly, and conversational speech contained a close to normal ratio of closed to open class words.

While the patient's poorer verbal agility scores suggest a new motor speech problem that might have given rise to the stuttering-like behavior, his improved auditory comprehension and word-finding ability suggest that the dysfluency might be associated with changes in his aphasia. Luchsinger and Arnold (1965) discuss a syndrome they call dysarthric stuttering, which may occur during the recovery phase of any type of aphasia. Although it has been linked most frequently in literature to recovery from anterior aphasias, patients with conduction aphasia, a posterior syndrome, often display stuttering-like behavior. This behavior may be a manifestation of their underlying problem with phonemic selection and ordering and their tendency to be highly self-critical of their errors. This explanation may hold also for the patient just described. He began to produce stuttering-like repetitions on the initial syllables of substantive words at the same time that he showed improvement in his ability to comprehend speech, to retrieve labels and to self-monitor his verbal output. Over the next few months, with continued language therapy, his aphasia decreased, and with it the stuttering-like behavior, making direct treatment of the dysfluency problem unnecessary.

Stuttering with Head Trauma

Stuttering may occur following trauma to the brain. The most common type of major brain trauma is closed head injury (CHI) resulting from motor vehicle accidents. The brain damage that follows sudden impact may be quite different from that caused by stroke. In CHI the brain may suffer focal damage due to compression of the skull, skull fractures with depressed bone fragments, or traumatic hemorrhages. In addition to focal damage, CHI may cause diffuse, microscopic damage to white matter pathways throughout the brain. This is diffuse axonal injury and may be associated with prolonged coma. Like stroke patients, it is not uncommon for CHI patients to develop seizure syndromes.

The overall neurological and neurobehavioral picture of CHI patients is typically more complicated than that of stroke patients. Among the behaviors common to CHI patients are memory problems, personality disorders, and dramatic changes in cognitive style with a loss of ability to think abstractly. In addition, the typical CHI patient is a young adult male who may have had a pretrauma history of reckless or irresponsible behavior and school problems (Levin, Benton, & Grossman, 1982). As with stroke patients who stutter, it is important to identify and delineate the presence and nature of any language impairment that might exist in CHI patients who stutter. Several factors may complicate evaluation of aphasia in CHI patients. Among these are the previously mentioned inattentiveness, memory loss, and concrete thinking with a tendency to quibble over answers. The reduction of cognitive levels after CHI may be a powerful obstacle to successful management of a posttraumatic stutter. CHI patients may be hampered by memory problems in retaining new material such as time and place of appointment, instructions, and therapeutic strategies. The level of motivation and concern of a CHI patient may be so low as to preclude a successful treatment program even if memory is intact. A patient with stuttering following CHI is described below.

A 32-year-old man was admitted to the Boston Veterans Administration Medical Center for a seizure disorder 7 years after an automobile accident in which he experienced a closed head injury. His pregnant wife was killed. Following the accident he was in a coma for about 4 days and awoke with a right hemiparesis and slurred speech that cleared in 2–3 weeks. About 3 years later he developed a seizure disorder and began to stutter. At the time of referral to the speech pathology department his seizures were poorly controlled and an EEG showed a left temporal abnormality. His speech was severely dysfluent with prolongations and repetitions occurring on virtually every syllable. Secondary characteristics such as clenching of fists, facial grimacing, and foot stamping were present. Despite BDAE scores in the nonaphasic range, his conversational speech tended to be telegraphic. This was probably due to "economy of effort" because he could produce fully grammatical sentences when encouraged to do so. Fluency was not facilitated by unison speaking, shadowing, or singing. Moments of fluency occurred only on recitation of the Lord's Prayer and subvocalizations during problem-solving tasks such as block designs.

His Wechsler Adult Intelligence Scale full scale verbal IQ was 93 and his performance IQ was 73. He experienced significant difficulty with object assembly, block designs, and visual memory tasks. Rhythmic tapping, repeated sequential hand movements, and three-dimensional drawings were poor. The patient entered a course of speech therapy that was interrupted frequently by periods of psychological withdrawal and medical problems, which eventually led to his transfer to another service. While on that service, about 4 months after hospital admission, he committed suicide.

Stuttering with Extrapyramidal Diseases

In 1971 Canter described several forms of neurogenic stuttering. Among these is what he refers to as "dysarthric stuttering" seen most often in patients with Parkinson's disease. This form is thought to be a result of faulty motor execution that gives rise to both slurred speech and sound prolongations, repetitions, and blocks associated with articulatory freezing. Sometimes the speech blocks are part of a general inability to initiate any motor activity. More recently, Koller (1983) described five Parkinson's patients whose stuttering occurred in the early stages of the disease. A sixth patient had gradual onset of stuttering for 1 year before other signs of progressive supranuclear palsy became evident. These cases confirm the association of stuttering with basal ganglia disease in some patients, although stuttering may be relatively rare in that population. When stuttering does occur in Parkinson's disease, however, its presence may represent a significant handicap for the patient. Two such patients, referred to the author, had only mild symptoms of Parkinson's disease except in the area of speech. One had good articulation but prominent stuttering-like behaviors. The other had stuttering associated with low volume and rapid speech rate. In both cases the speech problem prevented them from carrying on their jobs and motivated them to seek help from a speech pathologist when Levo-dopa failed to induce improvement. Similarly, Koller reports that the speech of his patients did not necessarily improve with Levo-dopa. A patient with Parkinsonian stuttering is described below.

> A 62-year-old man was referred to the speech pathology department with a 5-year history of gradually worsening stuttering and a 7-year history of micrographia. Two years prior to the speech referral he was seen by a neurologist, who found increased muscle tone, decreased facial expression, and some bradykinesia. Sinamet did not improve his speech. The stuttering continued to worsen and forced his retirement. Speech examination showed moderate to severe stuttering characterized by repetition of most initial and, occasionally, medial phonemes of both closed and open class words. Speech rate was rapid. Despite the dysfluencies he always persisted and finished his utterances. He verbally expressed

frustration but did not exhibit secondary motor characteristics. Neuropsychological testing showed him to have a Full Scale IQ of 148 (very superior range). He entered a course of speech therapy and responded positively to a pacing technique (described later in this chapter).

Stuttering with Tumor and Dementia

Another progressive disease that has been linked to adult-onset stuttering is dialysis dementia. At least three such cases have been documented in the literature (see Rosenbek, McNeil, Lemme, Prescott, & Alfy, 1975; and Madison et al., 1977). In these patients, who had undergone prolonged periods of dialysis for kidney disease, stuttering appeared with early signs of dementia and confusion. Later, the stuttering was replaced by intermittent mutism and, finally, mutism and death.

Recurrence of childhood stuttering was the first symptom of an Alzheimer's-like dementing process in a case described by Quinn and Andrews (1977). The stuttering occurred in a successful 62-year-old businessman 7 months before any other signs of disease. Seven months after onset, the stutter was so severe that he was referred again for treatment and found to have mild aphasia and cognitive losses. He experienced a steady downhill course and died 18 months after the onset of the first symptoms. Similarly, a 51-year-old man referred to the author had a 4-year history of increasing problems with memory and speech. His family characterized the initial speech problems as stuttering. When evaluated 4 years later, he was found to speak in short (2–3 words) empty phrases, for example, "these things" and "take to." He was very difficult to test because of severe problems in establishing "set." Auditory comprehension and naming seemed severely impaired, and he could not carry out tasks of reading and writing.

Severe stuttering developed in a 54-year-old woman with a metastatic brain tumor (Helm, Butler, & Canter, 1980). Although the first signs were an ataxic gait and right hyperreflexia, 3 weeks later she began to stutter on primarily the initial phonemes of both functor and substantive words. There was no adaptation effect. She deteriorated further neurologically and lapsed into mutism before death.

These cases once again make the point that onset of stuttering in a well-adjusted adult should be regarded as a possible symptom of neurological disease. Quinn and Andrews (1977) state that only in retrospect was it realized that their patient was making uncharacteristic errors of business judgment. The speech pathologist should stress to the physician that the stuttering may be symptomatic of a neurological disease and that a full workup is warranted, including a neuropsychological exam. This may be the major contribution made by the speech pathologist in cases of progressive dementia.

Stuttering with Drug Usage

Stuttering has been linked to the use of various pharmacological agents. Quader (1977) describes two cases in which administration of amitriptyline, a tricyclic antidepressant, resulted in stuttering speech. In both cases speech returned to normal when the drug was discontinued. A 4-year-old boy described by McCarthy (1981) developed severe stuttering every time theophylline (a broncho dialator) was administered for asthma. Nurnberg and Greenwald (1981) experienced difficulty in arriving at the correct dosages of a phenothiazine to control both psychosis and stuttering in two chronic patients with schizophrenia. With reduced drug levels the patients were fluent but psychotic. With higher levels the psychosis was controlled, but severe stuttering occurred.

Other Causes of Neurogenic Stuttering

In the previous sections the primary etiological classes of neurogenic stuttering were discussed. These findings are based largely upon published reports. This writer's clinical experience suggests that neurogenic stuttering may have still other causes. For example, a 48-year-old man who experienced brain anoxia during open heart surgery was referred to us for stuttering. His other neurobehavioral symptom was impaired memory. Another man with adolescent onset of seizures stuttered transiently after a suicide attempt involving dilantin overdose. A 16-year-old left-handed male with a childhood history of dystonia developed persistent severe stuttering and dysarthria following cryo-surgery to the right thalamus. The left thalamus had been treated earlier without speech changes. A 30-year-old electrician experienced transient stuttering (about 6 weeks duration) following inhalation of toxic fumes.

None of the patients mentioned above had a history of functional diseases or behaviors, so their stuttering was assumed to be neurologically based. That is not to say that hysterical or malingered stuttering is not ever a possibility in adults. For example, neurogenic stuttering was ruled out in one case seen by us because: (1) There was no known precipitating event, (2) there were no other neurological or neurobehavioral symptoms, (3) there was a positive history of psychogenic episodes, and

(4) the patient stood to gain from the speech disorder (it would force him to stop work and receive disability payments and early retirement).

DIAGNOSIS AND ASSESSMENT
OF NEUROGENIC STUTTERING

It is known that stuttering can arise in previously fluent adults after neurological damage or disease. Depending upon which brain struc-tures are involved, the neurological, speech, language, and neuropsychological characteristics of these individuals will differ. In the previous sections neurogenic stuttering was discussed according to broad etiological groupings, that is, stroke, head trauma, progressive diseases, and drug usage. In this section some suggested guidelines are provided for the diagnosis and assessment of this speech disorder. It should be understood, however, that the study of neurogenic stuttering is immature relative to the study of developmental stuttering, and these suggestions therefore are based upon incomplete evidence. In reviewing the evidence, however, an attempt was made to identify findings that have been reported by more than a single investigator and, therefore, appear robust. Only the characteristics of stroke, extrapyramidal disease, and head trauma patients are discussed because more information regarding the speech and neuropsychological profiles of these patients is available and because they are more likely candidates for treatment than patients with rapidly progressing diseases. After the characteristics of the three major diagnostic groups are described, suggestions are made for testing and identifying these behavioral features.

Characteristics of the Stroke-Induced Stutterer

Although more information is available regarding individuals who stutter following stroke than any other etiology, it is difficult to assemble a behavior profile of the typical stroke patient who stutters. This is partly because the published studies vary in the details reported and partly because the patients themselves vary along many dimensions: the cause of stroke, the number and the site(s) of stroke, the medical history, and the age at onset. The characteristics listed in this section (see Table 8.1) were compiled from numerous sources: Arend, Handzel, and Weiss (1962), Rosenfield (1972), Helm, Butler, and Benson (1978), Rosenbek, Messert, Collins and Wertz (1978), Donnan (1979), Mazzucchi et al. (1981), and Rosenfield, Miller, and Feltovich (1981). They are meant to

Table 8.1
"Typical" Characteristics of Stroke-Induced Stutterer (Usually Sudden in Onset)

Dysfluencies may be heard on	Initial phonemes (always)
	Medial phonemes (often)
	Substantive words (always)
	Functor words (often)
	Conversation (always)
	Repetition, automatized sequences, rote para-
	graphs, singing, and tapped speech (usually)
	There is no adaptation effect
Concomitant findings	Secondary motor signs (rare)
	Aphasia (sometimes)
	Bucco/facial apraxia (sometimes)
Often reduced performance in	"Carrying" a tune
	Tapping rhythms
	Block designs from model
	Stick designs from memory
	Sequential hand positions
	Three-Dimensional drawing

represent the "typical" patient with stroke-induced stuttering, although *typical* may not be a word to use when discussing any brain-damaged patient.

Characteristics of the Head Trauma–Induced Stutterer

The effects of head trauma perhaps are even less predictable than the effects of stroke. Strokes occur within the organization of the cerebral vascular system, but head trauma can occur to any part of the brain as well as diffusely within the brain. Patients who stutter following head trauma share some characteristics with stroke patients who stutter. A few distinguishing characteristics emerge from a review of the cases reported in Quinn and Andrews (1977), Helm, Butler, and Benson (1978), Helm, Butler, and Canter (1980), Tobin and Olsen (1980), Baratz and Mesulam (1981), Mazzucchi et al. (1981) (see Table 8.2).

In summary, the neurobehavioral features that best distinguish the stroke-induced from head trauma–induced stutterer are the following: Stuttering in the stroke patient is more likely to be sudden in onset than in the head trauma patient; the stroke patient is more likely to be aphasic; and the head trauma patient is somewhat more likely to have a seizure disorder, to show an adaptation effect, or to have secondary motor characteristics.

Table 8.2
"Typical" Characteristics of Stutterer with Head Trauma (May be Gradual in Onset)

Dysfluencies may be heard on	Initial phonemes (always)
	Medial phonemes (often)
	In conversation (always)
	Substantive words (often)
	Functor words (often)
	Repetition, automatized sequences and rote para-
	graphs, tapped speech and singing (usually)
	Adaptation effect is rare
Concomitant findings	Seizure disorder (sometimes)
	Secondary motor signs (sometimes)
	Aphasia (sometimes)
May have reduced performances in	"Carrying" a tune
	Tapping rhythms
	Block designs from model
	Sticks from memory
	Sequential hand position
	Three-dimensional drawing

Characteristics of the Stutterer with Extrapyramidal Disease

Much of what is known about the behavioral characteristics of the individual who stutters following onset of progressive extrapyramidal diseases comes from Koller's (1983) study. His findings concur with my own clinical experience with two Parkinson's patients with onset of stuttering (see Table 8.3).

In summary, the features that best distinguish the individual who stutters with extrapyramidal disease from those who stutter with stroke or head trauma is that onset in extrapyramidal disease is almost always gradual, and there is no aphasia or buccofacial apraxia. The extrapyramidal disease patient also is more likely to show an adaptation effect and stutter only on self-formulated speech and substantive words.

Examining for Neurogenic Stuttering

As stated previously, it is important to distinguish the motor speech aspects of stuttering from aphasic word retrieval or formulation problems. This is best done by administering a standardized aphasia test

Table 8.3
"Typical" Characteristics of Stutterer with Extrapyramidal Disease
(Usually Gradual in Onset)

Dysfluencies may be heard on	Initial phonemes (always) Medial phonemes (often) Substantive words (always) Functor words (sometimes) In conversation (always) In repetition, automatized sequences, rote para- graphs, tapped speech, and singing (sometimes) Adaptation effect may be seen
Concomitant findings	No secondary motor signs, aphasia, bucco/facial apraxia
Reduced performance in	"Carrying" a tune Tapping rhythms Sequential hand positions

such as the BDAE (Goodglass & Kaplan, 1972b). In the textbook that accompanies this exam (Goodglass & Kaplan, 1972a), suggestions are made for determining the presence and severity of bucco/facial apraxia.

Speech Samples

Once it has been determined that the patient's dysfluencies cannot be accounted for solely by aphasia, the speech problem may be examined more closely. The first step in this examination process is to obtain tape-recorded speech samples elicited under various conditions. First, a conversational sample is obtained in the manner suggested by the BDAE, with the clinician first eliciting social speech, for example, "Well, how are you today?" Then more propositional speech, for example, "What is your name and full address?" and, finally, strings of narrative speech, for example, "What happened to bring you here today?" Second, an expository speech sample is obtained by asking the patient to describe the activities portrayed in an action picture such as the BDAE cookie theft picture. Third, the patient is asked to read orally a standard passage containing all the sounds in the English language. Two such passages are "The Grandfather Passage" (Darley, Aronson, & Brown, 1975) and "The Rainbow Passsage" (Fairbanks, 1960). Multiple sequential readings are used to test for an adaptation effect. Fourth, the patient is asked to repeat 3–5 word phrases containing both functor and substantive words, for example, "She is here." "Planes fly faster than birds." Fifth, highly automatized speech tasks such as recitation of the days of the week, the alphabet and counting, completion of nursery rhymes such as "Mary Had a Little Lamb" or rote material such as the

Lord's Prayer are obtained. Sixth, the patient is asked to hum, then sing a familiar song. Finally, the effect of rhythmic tapping or speech is sampled by asking the patient to tap out and say the phrase "Shave and a haircut—two bits" five times. These tasks are outlined in Appendix 1.

The tape-recorded speech samples then may be analyzed for moments and types of dysfluencies, that is, whether a dysfluency occurred on an initial or medial phoneme, whether it took the form of a repetition, prolongation or block, and whether it occurred on closed class (functor) words (e.g., *the*) or open class (substantive) words (e.g., *book*). This analysis is performed for each of the speech tasks, and the results are used both for purposes of differential diagnosis and for judging severity of the disorder. The results of the speech analysis also might point the way toward procedures for managing the dysfluency problem.

Other Neurobehavioral Tasks

In addition to the presence of a seizure disorder, aphasia, and bucco/facial apraxia, several other behavioral characteristics help distinguish persons with neurogenic stuttering. During the speech tasks it is important to look for secondary motor signs such as fist clenching and facial grimacing. When testing the effect of singing upon the fluency disorder, it should be noted whether the patient can carry a tune. If stuttering on words is disruptive to singing then the patient should be asked to hum. Rhythmic hand tapping should be tested by asking the patient to repeat at least three different rhythms six times each (see BDAE for example). Sequential hand movements (e.g., fist, flat of hand, edge of hand) also should be repeated at least six times each with both hands, if possible. The Block Design subtest of the Wechsler Adult Intelligence Scale and the stick-design test suggested in the Goodglass and Kaplan (1972a) text are important in assessing visual/spatial and visual memory functions. Three-dimensional drawing ability is assessed by asking the patient to draw a solid block and a house both upon command and to copy. The presence and absence of these problems can be noted along with the dysfluencies on a summary sheet (see Appendix 1).

MANAGEMENT
OF NEUROGENIC STUTTERING

Whereas there is a small but convincing body of literature describing neurogenic stuttering, there is little describing treatment of this disorder. The information provided here, therefore, is based primarily upon the writer's own clinical experience and that of the speech pathology staff at the Boston Veterans Administration Medical Center.

Pacing Techniques

Of the seven cases of stroke-induced neurogenic stuttering described by Rosenbek et al., (1978) only one received treatment. According to the authors, this 53-year-old man with right parietal lobe damage was referred to their service 24 hours after the stuttering began. He was fluent after only six sessions of a treatment program that required him to slow his speech rate to approximately 50 words per minute by speaking one syllable at a time. While no mention is made of the use of rate-controlling devices such as a metronome, this writer's experience suggests that many neurogenic stutterers are unable to maintain slower, or syllable-by-syllable, speech in conversation without a pacing device. The best devices seem to be those that control speech with tactile pacing. A past report described such an instrument, which was used with a patient having severe palalalia following encephaletic Parkinson's disease (Helm, 1979). Palalalia is the rapid repetition of whole words and phrases, as distinguished from stuttering, which involves repetition, blocks, and prolongation of phonemes. For example, if asked his name, the patient with palalalia would repeat "my name, my name, my name, . . ." up to 30 times, in an increasingly rapid and decreasingly intelligible manner. He could not control this with a metronome, and when asked to tap his leg with his hand, both the tapping and speech accelerated and deteriorated. Through clinical experimentation, a pacing board was developed. This board has six multicolored squares and raised wooden dividers (see Figure 8.1). The patient taps his finger from square to square while speaking in a syllable-by-syllable manner (Helm, 1981). This instrument also has proved effective with two patients who acquired stuttering in association with Parkinson's disease and with the patient described earlier who stuttered following bilateral thalamic cryosurgery for dystonia.

Other smaller pacing devices may prove as effective as the pacing board and more convenient. For example, one Parkinson's patient was able to control his speech rate and stuttering with a toggle switch mounted on a small block of wood. He carried the device in his pocket and moved the switch back and forth as he spoke. In a 1983 issue of *ASHA* another pacing device was described (Pacing Devices Developed). This device is molded from Kay-splint material to fit over the patient's forefinger. Before molding, holes are punched in the material so that

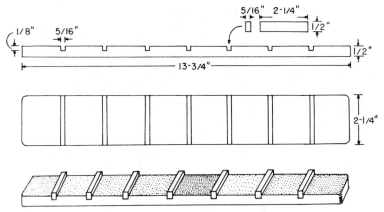

FIGURE 8.1   Pacing board.

the patient paces his or her speech by moving the thumb from hole to hole. Patients with tremor, however, may have difficulty using this device and may require the larger pacing board.

Delayed Auditory Feedback and Masking

In our clinic both a delayed auditory feedback (DAF) unit and Edinburgh Masker (Dewar, Dewar, Austin, & Brash, 1976) are available for trials with speech-disordered patients. Of the two devices, the Edinburgh masker appears more effective with neurogenic stuttering associated with rapid speech rates. Neither unit, however, has been more effective with our patients than pacing devices, which are less expensive by far. This is not to say that these instruments hold no therapeutic possibilities for neurogenic stutterers. Downie, Low, and Linsay (1981), for example, found DAF effective with 2 of 11 Parkinson's patients with speech disorders. One of the two had hesitations "akin to stammering." This suggests that DAF should be tried with neurogenic stutterers.

Transcutaneous Nerve Stimulation

Whereas patients who stutter with Parkinson's disease may have rapid but easy and seemingly effortless repetitions of phonemes, other neurogenic stuttering is slow and effortful. Such patients may show no improvement in fluency with pacing devices, DAE, or masking. A 1977 report by Helm and Butler described such a patient. This 68-year-old left-handed woman, who had been converted to her right hand for writing, had experienced a series of minor strokes to both cerebral hemispheres. Severe stuttering occurred after the fifth stroke, which also produced transient left hemiparesis. She had mild dysarthria and markedly dysfluent speech with severe blocking and prolongation of initial and medial syllables, especially consonant blends. Her language skills essentially were intact, but she had lost the ability to maintain pitch and melody, draw three-dimensional objects, and complete WAIS block designs. Trials with the pacing board *increased* dysfluencies. When an electro-larynx was vibrated against her left hand, moments of dysfluency in an oral reading task decreased from 38 to 8. A transcutaneous nerve stimulation (TNS) unit originally developed for control of pain proved similarly effective when applied to the bicipital groove of her left arm.

One of the problems encountered by clinicians who use TNS for treatment of pain is that the patient may habituate to the wave form so that the positive effects erode. This phenomenon seemed to be true in trials of TNS with other speech patients. This led to the development of a TNS unit with a variable wave form (Butler, Helm, & MacEachern, 1984). More clinical data is required before the effects of this TNS unit on neurogenic stuttering can be stated with any degree of certainty.

Biofeedback and Relaxation

Another approach to patients with effortful stuttering is based on the work of Kalotkin (1978), who experienced some success in treating 10 developmental stutterers by using biofeedback and relaxation. In this method, electrodes are placed over the masseter muscle bundles, and baseline tension levels are computed for 10 to 20 minutes of conversation and oral reading. The patient then is instructed in relaxation procedures while provided with visual (lights) and/or auditory (beeps or squeaks) feedback. By lowering masseter tension levels while talking, the patient can turn off the red light and/or sounds. Kalotkin's protocol is reproduced here with her permission (see Appendix 2).

One patient, so treated, had experienced onset of moderately severe stuttering after a series of small strokes. His articulation and grammar were normal in conversation, but he produced tense repetitions and blocks mostly on the initial sounds of words. There was no evidence of bucco/facial apraxia and his untimed WAIS performance IQ was 121. Using a Cyborg, BL 900 EMG Biofeedback Unit, an integrated (mean) masseter tension level of .61 μV was obtained for 5 minutes of conversation. He was given 5 minutes instruction in relaxation techniques, following which a mean tension level of .33 μV was obtained for 5 more minutes of conversation. He entered a 4-month, twice-weekly course of biofeedback/speech therapy with home practice in relaxation techniques and was only mildly dysfluent upon discharge.

A Parkinsonian stutterer failed to respond to this same program, pointing out once again that successful management of neurogenic stuttering requires differential treatment as well as differential diagnosis.

Pharmacological Agents

For some patients, one direction of treatment may be to explore with the patient's physician the effects of pharmacological agents on speech fluency. Dilantin levels, for example, may be associated with increased or decreased stuttering. Whereas we have seen stuttering with dilantin levels in the toxic range, Baratz and Mesulam's (1981) patient experienced diminished stuttering when seizures were brought under control with dilantin.

Haloperidol appears to have "a real, though limited, effect" on developmental stuttering in a positive direction (Bloodstein 1980, p. 355). This is a dopamine receptor blocking drug like the phenothiazides that caused stuttering in Nurnberg and Greenwald's (1981) two schizophrenic patients. To complicate the issue even further, amitriptyline, a drug that stimulates dopamine reception, caused stuttering in the two cases reported by Quader (1977), and theophylline, a catacholomine transmitter, induced stuttering in a 4-year-old child described by McCarthy (1981).

The only conclusion to be drawn at this time is that drugs that affect the basal ganglia may affect speech fluency in either a positive or negative direction. Careful, controlled drug trials may establish the correct levels for maintaining fluent speech in some patients.

SUMMARY

Adult onset neurogenic stuttering is a well-documented phenomenon that may occur with stroke, head trauma, progressive diseases, and drug use. Neurogenic stuttering is not a unitary disorder but will vary in its speech characteristics and associated neurobehavioral signs according to the etiology and site(s) of the brain lesion(s). Differential diagnosis will depend upon a careful examination which includes tests of aphasia, bucco/facial apraxia, and nonverbal motor and cognitive skills, as well as analysis of the stuttering during various speech tasks such as conversation, oral reading, repetition, and rote recitation. Neurogenic stuttering may be transient or persistent. For the persistent varieties several treatment approaches have been described. Among these are the use of speech pacing devices, delayed auditory feedback and masking, EMG biofeedback, and relaxation.

APPENDIX 1:
GUIDE TO DIFFERENTIAL DIAGNOSIS
OF NEUROGENIC STUTTERING

Speech Dysfluencies								
Speech Tasks	Initial phonemes			Medial phonemes			Functors	Substantives
	Block	Rep.	Prol.	Block	Rep.	Prol.		
Conversation								
Picture description								
Sentence repetition								
Reading −1								
(adaptation −2								
effect) −3								
Automatic Speech: Days of week								
Counting								
Passages								
Singing								
Tapped speech								
Concomitant findings								
	Present				Absent			
Aphasia								
Bucco/facial apraxia								

(continued)

Guide to Differential Diagnosis of Neurogenic Stuttering (*continued*)

	Concomitant findings	
	Present	Absent
Secondary motor signs		
Seizure disorder		
Poor tunes		
Poor rhythmic tapping		
Poor sequential hand positions		
Poor block designs		
Poor stick designs		
Poor 3-D drawings		

APPENDIX 2: KALOTKIN PROTOCOL: RELAXATION TRAINING FOR TREATMENT OF STUTTERING

Prefeedback

Step 1   Attach electrodes to masseter muscles of patient without allowing any feedback from machine.

Step 2   Integrate 10 min of conversation (have patient talk 10 min without feedback and prior to relaxation).

Step 3   Integrate five 1-min samples of oral reading.

Step 4   Integrate 10 min of relaxation (instruct patient to attempt to relax jaw muscles on his/her own).

Step 5   Read patient relaxation protocol: Instruct patient to practice protocol at home.

Feedback Stage

Step 1   Explain machine to patient, e.g., visual feedback (actual EMG level, binary), auditory modes.

Step 2   Test different auditory modes to judge which one seems most helpful to patient (1-min integrated levels).

Step 3   Choose auditory mode.

Step 4   Establish lowest relaxation level ($< 2.5 \mu V$).

CRITERION TO MOVE TO NEXT STEP
10-min integrated relaxation
level <2.5 μV

Step 5   Let patient observe feedback while he/she is speaking to establish a level of
EMG potential above which probability of blocking increases. Have patient
practice speaking keeping feedback off (feedback is now set so it only comes
on when dysfluency tension is reached). Intersperse this activity with other
training activities.

Step 6   Control over tension
Criteria to go to Next Task: Increase to specific μV level, hold for 10 sec (while
integrating), then alter to different μV level, etc. (integrated level within 10%
of goal μV).
a) Starting at relaxation threshold, increase to 3 μV, 6 μV, 8 μV, 10 μV, 30
μV, 60 μV, 100 μV.
b) Starting at 100 μV, follow the same progression down.
c) Random changes, up, down, large, small increments, i.e., 4 μV, 70 μV,
100 μV, 3 μV, 10 μV, 30 μV, 6 μV.

Step 7   Establish rapid relaxation threshold.
Criteria to Go to Next Task: Reach threshold within no more than 2 sec from
any given μV: 100 μV . . . relax, etc.

Step 8   Word Fluency Training (word or sentence depending on prior fluency level of
patient).
Patient must reach relaxation threshold before uttering word or phrase.
Criteria to Go to Next Task: For each list—1-min integrated without dysfluency.

Step 9   Establish hierarchy of speaking difficulty.
Situation: role-play using EMG feedback
Examples: 1.   reading
            2.   telephone
            3.   speaking to authority figures

Step 10 Continue conversational speech training with feedback. Shape to lowest level
that patient is able to speak and remain fluent.

Step 11 Integrate five 1-min samples of EMG tension during reading with feedback.

CRITERIA TO MOVE TO WEANING
10-min integrated conversation
2 μV less than baseline
No more than 5% dysfluency rate

Tape record sample of conversation and reading with feedback

Weaning Feedback

Wean feedback measure that gives patient least assistance first, then wean others (e.g.,
remove meter (visual), remove binary, then remove auditory).

Step 1 Establish relaxation
        Criteria 1. 1-min integrated level without feedback
               2.5 μV.
        Criteria 2. 10-min integrated level without feedback
               2.5 μV.
Step 2 Establish control over tension.
        a) high to mid to low level (10 sec integrated)
        b) low to mid to high (10 sec integrate)
        c) random
        (May have to backtrack and give some feedback to establish these levels). Clinician can at first tell patient when he/she has reached desired level; then patient can raise hand when he/she thinks he/she is at that level.
Step 3 Establish rapid relaxation threshold.
        (Same criteria as Step 7 with feedback)
        a) high (100 μV) to threshold
        b) mid (50 μV) to threshold
        c) low (4 μV) to threshold
Step 4 Fluency training
        Same as with feedback
        CRITERIA (Same as with Feedback without dysfluency 1 min).
Step 5 Integrate five 1-min samples of reading without feedback.

CRITERIA TO END TRAINING
10-min conversation without
feedback 2 μV from baseline
no more than 5% dysfluency

REFERENCES

Albert, M., Goodglass, H., Helm, N., Rubens, A., & Alexander, M. (1981) *Clinical aspects of Dysphasia*. New York: Springer-Verlag.

Arend, R., Handzel, L., & Weiss, B. (1962). Dysphatic stuttering. *Folia Phoniatria, 14,* 55–56.

Baratz, R., & Mesulam, M. (1981). Adult onset stuttering treated with anticonvulsants. *Archives of Neurology, 38,* 132.

Bloodstein, O. L. (1980). *Handbook of stuttering* (3rd ed.). Chicago: National Easter Seal Society.

Butler, R. B., Helm, N. H., & MacEachern, W. (1984). Transcutaneous Nerve Stimulator with Pseudo-random Pulse Generator, U.S. Patent #4,431,000.

Canter, G. (1971). Observations on neurogenic stuttering: A contribution to differential diagnosis. *British Journal of Disorders of Communication, 6,* 139–143.

Darley, F. L., Aronson, A. E., & Brown, J. R. (1975). *Motor speech disorders,* Philadelphia: Saunders.

Dewar, A., Dewar, A. D., Austin, W. T. S., & Brash, H. M. (1976). The long term use of an automatically triggered auditory feedback masking device in the treatment of stammering. *British Journal of Disorders of Communication, 14(3),* 219–229.

Donnan, G. A. (1979). Stuttering as a manifestation of stroke. *Medical Journal of Australia* 1: 44–45.

Downie, A. W., Low, J. M., & Linsay, D. D. (1981). Speech disorders in Parkinsonism: Use of delayed auditory feedback in selected cases. *Journal of Neurology, Neurosurgery, and Psychiatry, 44,* 852–853.

Fairbanks, G. (1960). *Voice and articulation drill book.* New York: Harper.

Farmer, A. (1975). Stuttering repetitions in aphasic and non-aphasic brain damaged adults. *Cortex, 11,* 391–396.

Goodglass, H., & Kaplan, E. (1972a). *The assessment of aphasia and related disorders.* Philadelphia: Lea and Febiger.

Goodglass, H., & Kaplan, E. (1972b). *Boston diagnostic aphasia exam.* Philadelphia: Lea and Febiger.

Helm, N. A. (1979). Management of palalalia with a pacing board. *Journal of Speech and Hearing Disorders, 44,* 350–353.

Helm, N. A. (1981). *Pacing boards.* Austin, TX: Exceptional Resources.

Helm, N. A., & Butler, R. B. (1977). Transcutaneous nerve stimulation in acquired speech disorder. *Lancet, 3,* 1177–1178.

Helm, N. A., Butler, R. B., & Benson, D. F. (1978). Acquired stuttering. *Neurology, 28,* 1159–1165.

Helm, N. A., Butler, R. B., & Canter, G. J. (1980). Neurogenic acquired stuttering. *Journal of Fluency Disorders, 5,* 269–279.

Kalotkin, M. (1978). *Electromyography in the treatment of stuttering.* Unpublished master's thesis, Emerson College, Boston.

Koller, W. C. (1983). Dysfluency (stuttering) in extrapyramidal disease. *Archives of Neurology, 40,* 175–177.

Levin, H. S., Benton, A. L., & Grossman, R. G. (1982). *Neurobehavioral consequences of closed head injury.* New York: Oxford University Press.

Luchsinger, R., & Arnold, G. E. (1965). *Voice-Speech-Language.* Belmont, CA: Wadsworth.

Madison, D., Baeher, E., Bazell, M., Hartman, K., Mahurkar, S. & Dunea, G. (1977). Communicative and cognitive deterioration in dialysis dementia. Two case studies. *Journal of Speech and Hearing Disorders, 42,* 238–246.

Manual of the International Statistical Classification of Diseases, Injuries & Causes of Death (Vol. 1). (1977). Geneva: World Health Organization.

Mazzucchi, A., Moretti, G., Carpeggiani, P., Parma, M. A., & Paini, P. (1981). Clinical observations in acquired stuttering. *British Journal of Disorders of Communication, 16,* 19–30.

McCarthy, M. M. (1981). Speech effect of theophylline. (Letter to the editors) *Pediatrics, 68,* 5.

Nurnberg, H. G., & Greenwald, B. (1981). Stuttering: An unusual side effect of phenothiazines. *American Journal of Psychiatry, 138,* 386–387.

Pacing Devices Developed. (1983). *ASHA, 25,* (4), 16.

Quader, S. E. (1977). Dysarthria: An unusual side effect of tricyclic antidepressants. *British Medical Journal, 9,* 97.

Quinn, P. T. & Andrews, G. (1977). Neurological stuttering: A clinical entity? *Journal of Neurology, Neurosurgery, Psychiatry, 40,* 699–701.

Raven, T. C. (1960). *Guide to the standard progressive matrices.* London: Lewis.

Rosenbek, J. C., McNeil, M. R., Lemme, M. L., Prescott, J. E., & Alfy, A. C. (1975). Speech and language findings in a chronic hemodialysis patient: A case report. *Journal of Speech and Hearing Disorders, 40,* 2.

Rosenbek, J., Messert, B., Collins, M. & Wertz, R. (1978). Stuttering following brain damage. *Brain and Language, 6,* 82–86.

Rosenfield, D. B. (1972). Stuttering and cerebral ischemia. *New England Journal of Medicine, 287,* 991.

Rosenfield, D. B., Miller, S. D., & Feltovich, M. (1981). Brain damage causing stuttering. *Transactions of the American Neurological Association, 105,* 1-3.

Tobin, H. W., & Olsen, B. D. (1980). Adult onset stuttering. *Journal of the Maine Medical Association, 71,* (1), 11-12.

Trost, J. (1971, November). *Apraxic dysfluency in patients with Broca's aphasia.* Paper presented at ASHA Convention, Chicago.

Wechsler, D. (1955). *The Wechsler adult intelligence scale.* New York: The Psychological Corporation.

Author Index

Numbers in *italic* refer to pages on which complete references are cited.

A

Ackerman, B. L., 160, *190*
Adams, M. R., 5, 7, 75, 76, 78, 86, *89, 90*
Albert, M., 195, *215*
Alexander, M., 195, *215*
Alfy, A. C., 201, *216*
Ames, S., 76, *90*
Anderson, V. A., 160, *188*
Andrews, G., 3, 7, 41, 52, *60*, 65, 72, 73, 76, *89, 152*, 155, 165, *188, 191*, 201, 204, *216*
Ansberry, M., 174, 180, *192*
Arend, R., 195, 203, *215*
Arnold, G. E., 155, 157, 161, 162, 163, 164, 166, 167, 168, 169, 172, 180, *188, 190*, 195, 198, *216*
Aronson, A. E., 206, *215*
Arsenian, J., 13, *33*
Ashmore, L. L., 107, *121*
Austin, W. T. S., 209, *215*

B

Baeher, E., 201, *216*
Bakwin, H ., 157, 161, 164, 169, *188*
Bakwin, R. M., 157, 161, 164, 169, *188*
Ballard, P. B., 127, *152*
Bandura, A., *188*
Baratz, R., 204, 211, *215*
Barbara, D. A., 93, 97, *121*

Bass, C., 137, *153*, 178, *190*
Bazell, M., 201, *216*
Benson, D, F., 194, 195, 203, 204, *216*
Benton, A. L., 198, *216*
Berdine, W. H., 125, *152*
Bernstein, L., 48, *60*
Bernstein, R., 48, *60*
Berry, M. F., 164, 165, *188*
Berryman, J., 40, 41, *61*
Bialer, J., 128, *154*
Blackhurst, A. E., 125, *152*
Blaesing, L., 76, *89*
Blood, G. W., 174, *188*
Bloodstein, O., 3, 7, 13, *33*, 35, 38, 39, *60*, *61*, 65, *89*, 95, 96, 99, 105, *121*, 126, 129, 137, *152*, 159, 165, *188*, 211, *215*
Bluemel, C. S., 166, *188*
Boberg, E., 76, *89*, 126, 127, *152*
Boland, J. L., 101, *121*
Bonfanti, B. H., 129, 130, 132, *152*
Bradford, D., 180, 181, *188*
Bradwick, J., 41, *61*
Brady, W. A., 126, 127, *152*
Brash, H. M., 209, *215*
Brayton, E. R., 131, *153*
Breen, K., 179, *189*
Brown, J. R., 206, *215*
Brownmiller, S., 43, 45, *60*
Brutten, E. J., 66, *89*
Bryne, B. M., 107, *121*
Bullen, A. K., 14, *33*

219

Butler, R. B., 194, 195, 201, 203, 204, 210, 215, 216

Downie, A. W., 209, 216
Dunea, G., 201, 216

C

Cabanas, R., 130, 132, 152, 163, 168, 188
Calvert, J. J., 170, 192
Campbell, S., 49, 61
Canter, G., 195, 201, 204, 215, 216
Carpeggiani, P., 195, 203, 204, 216
Carr, A., 174, 180, 192
Carter, D., 181, 189
Chapman, A. H., 127, 129, 132, 152
Chappel, C. R., 160, 190
Chess, S., 110, 122
Clark, W., 41, 62
Clifton, Jr., N. F., 130, 154
Cole, J., 81, 91
Collins, M., 155, 191, 195, 203, 208, 216
Conture, E. G., 3, 4, 7, 175, 176, 182, 188
Cooper, C. S., 137, 138, 143, 144, 146, 153
Cooper, E. B., 42, 60, 127, 129, 132, 137, 138, 139, 140, 143, 144, 146, 149, 152, 153, 175, 182, 188
Costa, L. D., 178, 188
Cox, M. D., 95, 96, 99, 101, 102, 103, 106, 108, 109, 122
Craig, A., 3, 6, 7, 65, 89
Cruickshank, W. M., 172, 188
Culatta, R., 129, 130, 132, 152
Cullinan, W. L., 75, 89, 129, 154
Cutler, J., 41, 60, 72, 73, 89

D

Dahlstrom, W. G., 105, 121
Dalton, P., 155, 156, 169, 174, 189
Daly, D. A., 4, 7, 104, 122, 137, 153, 155, 160, 166, 172, 174, 176, 177, 178, 179, 181, 183, 189, 190, 191
Dana, R., 48, 60
Darley, F. L., 69, 75, 89, 90, 206, 215
Darnton, S. W., 176, 178, 189
de Ajuriaguerra, J., 168, 190
de Hirsch, K., 157, 162, 165, 189
Despert, J. L., 107, 109, 121
Dewar, A., 209, 215
Dewar, A. D., 209, 215
Donnan, G. A., 203, 215
Douglass, E., 39, 60

E

Edson, S. K., 126, 153
Erickson, R. L., 41, 60, 72, 89, 178, 189
Evans, D., 48, 60
Ewart, B., 126, 127, 152

F

Fairbanks, G., 206, 216
Falck, F. J., 157, 189
Farber, N., 178, 188
Farmer, A., 131, 153, 195, 216
Feltovich, M., 203, 217
Fenichel, O., 97, 121
Feyer, A. M., 3, 7, 65, 89
Fiscus, E., 125, 153
Florance, C. L., 181, 184, 186, 189, 191
Fraiberg, S., 46, 60
Freeman, F. J., 174, 189
Freund, H., 156, 160, 164, 172, 189
Frick, J. V., 190
Fristoe, M., 177, 190
Froeschels, E., 157, 162, 163, 165, 169, 172, 179, 190
Froseth, J. O., 178, 189

G

Gaines, T., 54, 61
Gendleman, E. G., 78, 89
Gilligan, C., 53, 60
Gladstein, K., 36, 41, 42, 61
Glasner, P. J., 37, 60, 107, 109, 110, 121
Glauber, I. P., 93, 97, 121
Gleason, J. R., 4, 7
Godenne, G., 53, 60
Goldman, R., 77, 89, 177, 190
Goldstein, A., 78, 90
Goodglass, H., 195, 196, 205, 206, 207, 215, 216
Goodstein, L. D., 99, 103, 105, 121
Gordon, M. M., 11, 33
Gottsleben, R. H., 126, 127, 128, 132, 153, 154
Gove, P. B., 192
Gray, M., 43, 60

Greenwald, B., 202, 211, *216*
Gregory, H. H., 166, 175, 182, *190*
Grewel, F., 163, *190*
Grossman, H. J., 124, 125, *153*
Grossman, R. G., 198, *216*
Guitar, B., 6, 7, 52, *60*, 72, 74, 76, *89*, 137, *153*, 178, *190*
Gutzmann, Sr., H., 159, 169, *190*

H

Hall, D. E., 126, 127, *152*
Halls, E. C., 127, *153*
Handzel, L., 195, 203, *215*
Hardcastle, W. J., 155, 156, 169, 174, *189*
Hardyck, C., 77, *89*
Harris, M., *152*, 165, *188*
Hartman, K., 201, *216*
Hathaway, S. R., 101, *121*
Healey, E. C., 76, *90*
Healey, W. C., 160, *190*
Hearn, M., 48, *60*
Hecaen, H., 168, *190*
Helm, N. A., 194, 195, 201, 203, 204, 208, 210, *215*, *216*
Helmreich, H., 39, *61*
Henley, N., 53, 56, *62*
Herskovits, M. J., 9, 30, *33*
Hill, D., 166, 175, 182, *190*
Hinzman, A. R., 160, *191*
Hoddinott, S., 3, 7, 65, *89*
Hood, S. B., 175, *190*
Horynak, A., 52, *61*
Howie, P., 3, 6, 7, 52, *60*, 65, 76, *89*
Hunt, J., 157, *190*

I

Ierodiakonou, C. S., 107, 110, *121*
Ingham, R. J., 5, 6, 7, 76, *90*
Irvine, T. L., 160, 171, 180, 183, 188, *192*
Ivey, A., 48, *60*
Ivey, M., 41, *61*

J

Jacklin, E., 53, *61*
Johns, J. S., 172, *188*
Johnson, W., 14, *34*, 35, 38, 39, 40, 41, 43, *61*, 66, 69, 75, *90*, 160, *188*

Jonassen, S., 176, *189*
Jones, E., *121*

K

Kalotkin, M., 210, *216*
Kanfer, F., 78, *90*, 181, *190*
Kaplan, E., 195, 196, 205, 206, 207, *216*
Karlin, I. W., 127, *153*
Keane, V. E., 127, *153*
Kelly, J. S., 76, *90*
Kidd, J., 71, *90*
Kidd, K., 36, 41, 42, *61*, 71, *90*, 185, *189*, *190*
Kilburn, K. L., 126, 127, *154*
Kirk, S. A., 184, *190*
Kirk, W. D., 184, *190*
Kohut, H., 98, *121*, 122
Koller, W. C., 200, 205, *216*
Kools, J., 38, 39, 40, 41, *61*, 62
Kopp, G. A., 160, *188*
Kraemer, C., 56, *61*

L

Landolt, H., 170, *190*
Langford, W. S., 157, 164, 165, 166, 183, *189*
Langova, J., 157, 170, 174, 182, *190*
Lankford, S. D., 139, *153*
Lass, N., 65, *90*
Leavitt, R. R., 10, 13, *34*
Lehrman, J. W., 77, *91*
Leininger, M., 9, 30, *34*
Leith, W. R., 17, 24, *34*
Lemme, M. L., 201, *216*
Lerman, J. W., 128, *153*
Levin, H. S., 198, *216*
Levita, E., 178, *188*
Lewis, D., 75, *90*
Lezak, M. D., 178, *190*
Liebetrau, R. M., 155, *190*
Liebmann, A., 159, 163, 169, *190*
Lindsay, K., 126, 127, *152*
Linsay, D. D., 209, *216*
Lohr, F., 4, 7
Louttit, C. M., 127, *153*
Low, J. M., 209, *216*
Lubman, C. G., 126, *153*

Luchsinger, R., 161, 162, 166, 167, 168, 169, 170, 180, *190*, 195, 198, *216*
Lynch, J., 50, 54, *61*

M

McCarthy, J. J., 184, *190*
McCarthy, M. M., 202, 211, *216*
Maccoby, E., 53, *61*
MacEachern, W., 210, *215*
McEneaney, J., 77, *91*
McKinely, J. C., 101, *121*
McLelland, J. K., 139, 140, *153*
McNeil, M. R., 201, *216*
Madison, D., 201, *216*
Mahurkar, S., 201, *216*
Mallard, A. R., 76, *90*
Mandell, C. J., 125, *153*
Maning, W. H., 88, *90*
Martyn, M. M., 42, *61*, 126, 127, *153*, *154*
Mase, D. J., 160, *188*
Mason, G., 126, 127, *152*
Mazzuchi, A., 195, 203, 204, *216*
Mehrabian, A., 48, *61*
Messert, B., 155, *191*, 195, 203, 208, *216*
Mesulam, M., 204, 211, *215*
Metz, D., 75, *90*
Meyer, V., 76, *90*
Miller, S. D., 76, *90*, 203, *217*
Mims, H. A., 17, 24, *34*
Mishler, C., 179, *189*
Moncur, J. P., 109, 110, *121*, *122*
Montgomery, A., 39, *61*
Moore, W. H., 155, *190*
Moravek, M., 157, 170, 174, 182, *190*
Moretti, G., 195, 203, 204, *216*
Morgenstern, J. J., 17, *34*
Morley, M. E., 164, *191*
Morse, W. C., 172, *188*
Myers, G., 48, *61*
Myers, J., 52, *61*
Myers, M., 48, *61*

N

Naroll, R., 14, *34*
Naylor, R. V., 75, *90*
Neilson, M., 3, *7*, 65, *89*

Novak, A., 156, 162, 164, *191*
Nurnberg, H. G., 202, 211, *216*

O

Oakes, K., 179, *189*
Olsen, B. D., 204, *217*
Op't Hof, J., 160, *191*
Ostreicher, H., 176, *189*
Otto, F. M., 131, *153*
Owen, N., 84, 85, *90*

P

Packman, A., 76
Paini, P., 195, 203, 204, *216*
Parma, M. A., 195, 203, 204, *216*
Pearson, L., 159, 163, 178, *191*
Peins, M., 78, *90*
Perkins, W. H., 67, 75, 80, 85, *90*
Perrin, K. L., 160, *190*
Petrinovich, L., 77, *89*
Pizzat, F. J., 101, *122*
Powers, G. R., 128, *153*
Prather, E. M., 75, *89*
Prescott, J. E., 201, *216*
Preus, A., 4, *7*, 130, 132, *153*, *191*
Prins, D., 96, *122*
Prosek, R., 39, *61*
Purtilo, R., 30, *34*

Q

Quader, S. E., 202, 211, *216*
Quarrington, D., 108, *122*
Quarrington, B., 39, *60*
Quinn, P. T., 155, *191*, 201, 204, *216*

R

Raven, T. C., 197, *216*
Records, M., 71, *90*
Reis, R. P., 160, 171, 180, 183, 188, *192*
Rentschler, G. J., 3, *7*, 172, 178, *191*
Resnick, P., 76, *90*
Richmond, L., 54, *61*
Rigrodsky, S., 128, *153*
Riley, G. D., 4, *7*, 65, 68, 69, 75, *90*, 139, *153*, 166, 175, 176, 177, 182, *191*

Riley, J., 4, 7, 155, 166, 175, 176, 177, 182, 191
Robbins, S. D., 107, 122
Roman, K. G., 167, 191
Rosenbek, J. C., 155, 191, 195, 201, 203, 208, 216
Rosenfield, D. B., 93, 122, 191, 203, 217
Rosenthal, D., 37, 60
Rotter, J. B., 109, 122
Rubens, A., 195, 215
Rudolph, S. R., 88, 90
Ruggiero, A., 77, 91
Runyan, C. M., 75, 86, 89
Ryan, B. P., 5, 7, 66, 69, 90

S

Sacco, P., 75, 90
St. Louis, K. O., 65, 90, 160, 191
St. Onge, K. R., 4, 7, 170, 192
Saltz, E., 49, 61
Santostefano, S., 103, 122
Sasanuma, S., 38, 61
Schaeffer, M., 127, 153
Schiavetti, N., 75, 90
Schlanger, B. B., 127, 128, 132, 153, 154
Schnell, H., 160, 188
Schofield, W., 116, 122
Schubert, O. W., 126, 154
Schuell, H., 37, 43, 45, 61
Schwartz, D., 39, 61
Schwartz, H. D., 4, 7
Schwartz, M. F., 80, 90
Seeman, M., 156, 161, 162, 164, 191
Seider, R., 36, 41, 42, 61, 174, 188
Semour, C., 77, 91
Senekjian, M. A., 116, 122
Sermas, C. E., 95, 96, 99, 101, 102, 103, 106, 108, 109, 116, 122
Sewell, W. R., 88, 90
Shames, G. H., 181, 184, 186, 189, 191
Shearer, W., 42, 61, 127, 153
Sheehan, J. G., 35, 40, 41, 42, 49, 55, 61, 96, 99, 103, 122, 126, 127, 153, 154, 157, 191
Shepherd, G., 162, 163, 191
Sherman, D., 75, 90
Shine, R. E., 66, 91, 175, 182, 191

Shoemaker, D. J., 66, 89
Shover, J., 160, 188
Silverman, E. M., 36, 37, 39, 40, 41, 43, 45, 49, 51, 52, 53, 54, 60, 61, 62, 73, 91
Silverman, F., 38, 39, 40, 41, 62
Simon, C. A., 181, 189
Sitler, R., 75, 90
Skotko, D., 49, 61
Slutz, K., 126, 127, 153
Smith, A., 4, 7, 104, 122, 160, 177, 178, 179, 189, 191
Snidecor, J. C., 14, 34
Soderberg, G. A., 68, 70, 91
Spadino, E. J., 167, 191
Spradley, J. P., 30, 34
Spriestersbach, D., 69, 75, 90
Stark, R., 127, 154
Stewart, R., 181, 191
Stormer, J., 160, 190
Strazzulla, M., 127, 153
Sugarman, M., 52, 62

T

Tachell, R. H., 77, 91
Tanner, S., 76, 89
Tate, M. W., 129, 154
Thomas, A., 110, 122
Thompson, J., 178, 192
Thorn, K. F., 101, 122
Thorne, B., 53, 56, 62
Thorpe, L., 41, 62
Tiegs, E., 41, 62
Tiger, R. J., 160, 171, 180, 183, 188, 192
Tobin, H. W., 204, 217
Toplin, M., 98, 122
Trost, J., 195, 217
Tudor, M., 43, 44, 62

U

Uhlemann, M., 48, 60
Uys, I. C., 160, 191

V

VanDen Berg, 77, 91
Van Kirk Ryan, B., 5, 7
Van Opens, K., 37, 43, 45, 60, 62

Van Riper, C., 4, *8*, 13, *34*, 76, 78, *91*, 126,
    127, 133, 139, *154*, 156, 157, 166, 172,
    174, 183, *192*
Vaughan, G. H., 178, *188*
Versteegh-Vermeij, E., 50, *62*

W

Walden, B., 39, *61*
Wallen, V., 109, *122*
Walnut, F., 101, 102, *122*
Webster, R. L., 5, *8*, 76, *91*
Wechsler, D., 177, *192*, 197, *217*
Weiss, B., 195, 203, *215*
Weiss, D. A., 132, 133, *154*, 156, 157, 158,
    159, 160, 161, 163, 164, 165, 167, 168,
    169, 172, 173, 174, 175, 178, *188*, *192*
Wendell, R. W., 81, *91*
Wendiggensen, R., 76, *90*
Wertz, R., 155, *191*, 195, 203, 208, *216*
West, R., 174, 180, *192*
Willerman, L., 107, *121*
Williams, D. E., 38, 39, 50, *62*, 75, *89*,
    175, *192*

Williams, J., 42, *61*
Wingate, M. E., 42, *63*, 66, 67, 79, *91*, 172,
    192
Wohl, M. T., 127, *154*, 158, 161, *192*
Wolfe, W. G., 160, *188*
Woolf, G., 178, *192*
Wyatt, G. L., 104, *122*, 156, 157, *192*
Wynn, S., 126, 127, *152*

Y

Yairi, E., 43, 49, *63*, 130, 131, *153*, *154*
Yalom, I., 119, *122*

Z

Zelen, S., 35, 40, 41, *61*
Zimmer, C. H., 36, 37, 40, 41, 45, 51, 52,
    53, 54, 60, *62*, 73, *91*
Zimmerman, G., *63*, 80, *91*
Zisk, P. K., 128, *154*
Zwitman, D., 50, *63*

Subject Index

A

Abnormality
  articulation, 162
  breathing, 162
  phonation, 162
Acquired stuttering, *see* Neurogenic
  stuttering
Adaptation, 129
Alzheimer's disease, 201
Aphasia, 195
Articulation, clutterer, 176
Attention span, 159
Attitude, 40, 141
  clutterer, 178
  speech, 13
Atypical stutterer
  influence, cultural, 16, 18
  universality, 3, 30, 36
Awareness, 159

B

Biofeedback, 118

C

Case history, cluttering, 175
Cause
  cultural belief, 15
  diagnosogenic theory, 43
  environmental stress, 43
  neurogenic stuttering, 194
  parental attitudes, 108
  psychological trauma, 106–108
  alcohol abuse, 108
Central Language Imbalance, 157
Child rearing, 14, 97
Chronicity assessment, 139
Clinician
  characteristics, 6
  clinical needs, 33
  competency, 48
  stereotype, 36, 56
  training, 88, 160
  cluttering, 160
Closed head injury, 198
Cluttering
  definition, 156
  mentally retarded, 128, 130, 132, 168
  prevalence, 160
  prognosis, 183
  symptoms, 159–172
  facultative, 161
  obligatory, 159
  vs. learning disability, 171
  vs. stuttering, 132, 156, 161, 166, 171,
    172, 187
Consistency, 129
Conversion symptom, 97

Cortical stuttering, *see* Neurogenic stuttering
Counseling
  elementary school, 51
  preschool, 49
Culture, 9
  assimilation, 12
  authority, 19, 25, 27
  belief, 21, 29
  child rearing, 28
  eye contact, 26
  fluency, 23
  General American, 10
  gesture, 26
  impoliteness, 27
  incidence, 13, 14
  influence, 30–32
  male–female role, 16, 17, 20, 22, 25, 46, 56
  physical contact, 23
  privacy, 21
  resources, 29
  ritual, 22
  stress, 13, 14, 17, 45
  time orientation, 18, 24

D

Delayed auditory feedback, 171
Diagnosis, 18–23, 74–75, 110–114, 134–143, 175–179, 203–207
  adolescent, 52
  anxiety, 112
  depression, 112
  individualized, 45
  interviewing, 111
Dilantin, 211
Disfluency, 38
Disfluency Descriptor Digest, 149
Down's syndrome, 126, 130
Drugs, anxiety, 118
Dysarthric aphasia, 198

E

Electroencephalogram, 170
Elision, 162
Embolus, 194

Etiology, *see* Cause
Evil eye, 21
Expectancy, 129

F

Female, communication, 54
Female stutterer
  attitudes, 73
  data, 35
  group interaction, 53, 56
  menstrual cycle, 41
  recovery, 42
  referral, 37
  stereotype, 36, 46
  symptoms, 40
  therapy, 36
    effectiveness, 41, 42
    time after onset, 37, 42
  therapy preference, 53, 54
Fluency-initiating gesture, 146–149, 182

H

Haloperidol, 211
Hemorrhage, 194
Heredity, 169
Hyperactivity, 164

I

Implosion therapy, 78
Instrumentation, 148
Intelligence, 168
Interviewing
  elementary school, 50
  preschool, 47

M

Maintenance
  life-style, 84

L

Language, 165

recycling, 85
self-esteem, 84
Maladjusted stutterer
  child, 105
  definition, 94
  identification, 111
  origin, 106
  prevalence, 95
  team approach, 114
Maladjustment, 94
  child abuse, 108
  risk among stutterers, 100
Mental retardation
  classification, 124
  definition, 124
  deinstitutionalization, 149
  incidence, 126
  prevalence, 125
  services for, 134
Mentally retarded stutterer, 133
  attitudes, 137
  emotions, 145
  prevalence, 126
  symptoms, 128
  therapy, 136, 143, 145, 147
    group, 147
    group vs. individual, 149
    need for, 136
Minnesota Multiphasic Personality Inventory, 101
Monotony, 163
Motor ability, 164
Musical ability, 163

N

Neurogenic stuttering
  brain tumor, 201
  dementia, 201
  drug usage, 202
  extrapyramidal disease, 200, 205
  head trauma, 198, 204
  stroke, 194, 203
  types, 193
  vs. aphasia, 195
  word retrieval, 196
Neuropsychological assessment, 177, 207
Neurosis, 98

O

Organization of thought, 164

P

Pacing board, 208
Palalalia, 208
Parent
  adjustment, 105
  attitudes, 140
Parent–child interaction
  observation, 49
Parent–child relationship, 98
  sibling position, 109
Parkinson's disease, 200
Perceptual abilities, 160
Personality, 96, 169
Personalized Fluency Control Therapy–
    Revised (PFCT-R)
  diagnostic, 138–143
  therapy, 143–149
Projective techniques, 102
Proprioceptive awareness, 79
Prosody, 75
Psychoanalytic theory, 96
Psychological adjustment, 41
Psychological maladjustment, 94, see also
    Maladjustment
Psychological tests, 101
Psychotherapy, 114
  family therapy, 119
  group therapy, 118
  supportive, 115

R

Rate, see also Tachylalia
  festinating, 161
  rapid, 161
Rate of speech, 75
Reading, 167
Referral, 111
Repetition, 159
Research, 60
  needs, 123, 179, 187
Researcher, 33
  characteristics, 6
Rorschach test, 103

S

Self-concept, 109
Severe stutterer
  attitudes, 72
  handedness, 70
  inheritance, 70
  prevalence, 68
  prosody, 74
  rate of speech, 74
  sex ratio, 70
  symptoms, 67
  therapy, integrated approach, 76
Severity
  frequency fallacy, 137
  measures, 75
Sex ratio, 35, 36
  problems, 38
Spelling, 167
Stress, 80
Stress management, 117
Stroke, 194
Stutter-Free Speech Program, 181, 184, 186
Stuttering
  definition, 38, 66
  distribution, 39
  overlap with disfluency, 39
  symptoms, 140
    assessment, 140–143
Subculture, 11
  Hispanic, 10
Subgroup, 12, 94, 100, 120, 166, 172
  Van Riper tracks, 4
Summer Residence Stuttering Clinic, 69, 76–87
  dismissal, 86
  exposure, 77
  general explanation, 77
  highlighting, 81
  modification, 79
  rate of speech, 80
  stabilization and transfer, 79
Supportive personnel, 151
Symptoms, 38, 39, 66, 77

T

Tachylalia, 157, 161
Teachers, 140
Testing
  elementary school, 50
  preschool, 49
Thematic Apperception Test, 104
Therapy, 23–29, 53–59, 76–88, 114–120, 143–151, 179–187, 207–211
  biofeedback, 210
  communication skills, 56
  delayed auditory feedback, 209
  drug, 200, 211
  Edinburgh masker, 209
  effectiveness, 33
  failure, 85
  motivation, 83, 86
  pacing, 208
  role of practice, 148
  slow rate, 180
  standardized, 5
  stress reduction, 80
    hierarchy, 81
  transfer, 114
  transference, 113
Thrombosis, 194
Tranquilizer, 118
Transcutaneous nerve stimulation, 210
Treatment
  delayed auditory feedback, 182
  drug, 171
  interdisciplinary, 172
  multidisciplinary, 120
Typical stutterer, 3, 66, 95, 99
  definition, 193
  psychological profile, 104

V

Vowel stop, 163

W

Writing, 167
Word-finding problems, 165